THE MIND GAP

TO HAPPINESS

Master your thoughts and be happy

The ultimate practical guide towards a personal transformation. Understand your nature, find self-love and overcome worry, fear and anxiety.

To Egypt and all my Masters.

TABLE OF CONTENTS

INTRODUCTION

How many times have you tried to make resolutions in order to change your life and failed? Do ever find yourself questioning why you are unable to commit and to see the completion of any project you start? Are you dealing with anxiety and fear? Do you sometimes get overcome by feelings or thoughts that you cannot understand? Do you feel worrisome, lost and with no goals? If these questions have been running through your mind and you want to put an end to the cycle and stop being ruled by indecision, fear and anxiety so you can take control of your life, then this is the book for you.

In this book you will discover how to close the gap in your mind that stops you from moving forward and live a successful life. Learn how to recognize your own mind gap and close it, so you can finally be genuinely happy and enjoy your life.

The explanations in this book will help you understand how your mind, and the mind of others work, enabling you to start on your path to decluttering yourself of whatever has been stopping you from accomplishing your goals, and boost your willpower. Whether you want to achieve weight loss, your dream job, find your soul mate, or get out of debt, it all comes back to understanding your thought patterns and mindset. Find the true version of you as you take control over your life. This is a personal journey that only you can commit to undertake. If you don't, you will keep making the same mistakes. You may set out to accomplish new goals, maybe even convince yourself that you have a new mindset, but without working on yourself as it is shown in this book, everything you set out to accomplish will inevitably fail. You need to stop feeling troubled by negative emotions and feelings, and start understanding your thoughts. This book will show you how you can recalibrate your mind and develop positive habits for permanent change to get out of the vicious cycle of defeat.

Thousands of books have been published on motivation, dieting, mindfulness, and even biographies of people that have made it before you, but what they are not telling you is the secret to getting it done and unlock your destiny. The secret to your own success starts with you not interfering with your plans. Unless you understand yourself the tricks, fears, or longings, you have nothing you try will work. This is the only truth. In this book, you will find elaborate explanations with examples and practical exercises that allow you to explore your feelings and thoughts, understand them, and not get lost in them. It is imperative that you know yourself, your virtues and failures, accept them and move forward to a brighter future. This book is practical in offering you advice on how you can improve your life by understanding yourself and eventually attaining any goal you want to set on. Take a step into making your life easier, balanced and happier. You do not need to have any special gifts, we all have the potential to become our best self. The only way to start is by understanding all that is written in this book and practice the proposed exercises. Filled with powerful truths, thought-provoking activities, inspirational quotes, and lifestyle tips, this book will help you to find yourself and empower you to ultimately create the best version of you, so you can live in abundance. This is the key to find your own way in life and free yourself of anything that procrastinates you from becoming what you are meant to be. Stop feeling lost and take the courage to move forward, free yourself from your past, your fear and doubts, your dissatisfaction in live and your unhappiness. Don't give up on yourself, understand and tame your thoughts in a playful way as it is explained in this book. Try it, because only by trying new things you can get new results. This is the best of times to start. Take courage to become responsible for your happiness and do it today! I promise you will not regret it.

"Know thyself"

Temple of Apollo

CHAPTER ONE

KNOW YOURSELF

Y ou may feel the need to change and not know how to start or when you do, you find yourself being unable to stick with change. Self-defeating behavior is a common reason that prevents you from achieving the love, success and happiness you want in your live.

Know yourself, your unconscious thoughts and reactions, and stop sabotaging yourself and take the steps of action to transform your thoughts from self-defeating to life-enhancing ones.

One of the most important things you can do in life is to understand yourself. It is you who lives your life. You have to start making a personal evaluation of who you are and what areas of yourself are slowing and stopping you that need to be changed. First you need to declutter yourself. Many people think clutter is only of the physical things that surrounds us, but the first thing to clutter is your own mind. Physical clutter will cause us stress and anxiety, but it also can be due or cause of the clutter in our minds. You may not notice that you are not in control of your mind, neither your personal body. An important part of the journey of self-discovery is to understand with objectivity who you are and what affects and controls your life.

Have you ever found yourself questioning things you have done and not understanding why you did them? Why did you argue with your spouse and what were you arguing about in the first place? Why are you still in the same old job or love? Why have you been unable to reach your goals? Why you always give up? You have to know that our behavior is largely controlled by our subconscious, hence it is important that you comprehend why you make certain decisions or have certain reactions. However, if you understand how to look inside your thoughts, you can find greater knowledge about yourself as well as the answers to why you behave in a certain way, which are your fears, why you keep hanging on your sorrows, what causes you joy, and how to improve and change what you do not like about yourself.

You can start this journey to your real self-discovery, taking a personality test. There are different personality tests that you can take and you can find in internet. Just chose one and take it. Do it in a playful and inquiring way. When you get the results, do not take them too seriously, but ask yourself whether what they say about you is true. Remember that self-examination is the only way to awake your awareness of your own self.

The following pointers will guide you into the journey of finding out who you really are. Again, do it with ease, take it as an adventure into yourself. Learn what they say about you and if you think is right.

Objective Assessment

As I said before, there are several certified tests that you can take in order to understand different angles of yourself. It is important to find an objective assessment because of the biases that people around you hold about you and you may not get an accurate assessment of yourself. An objective assessment will give you a more accurate picture and help you consider things you never thought about. Here are the recommendations of tests you can look for:

- The Personality type theory by Myers-Briggs stipulates that a person has

1 of 16 basic personalities. These personalities are able to predict how you interact with people, your interpersonal challenges and strengths, and the best environment you are suited for. You can find this test online should you desire to do it.

- A career test is also advisable if you struggling to understand what makes you happy and what to do with your life. The tests help you establish what you find most satisfying based on your personality and hobbies. There are different types of career tests online to help you with this.

- Learning Style is a theory that says that each person learns and understands their experiences differently. Understanding your learning style helps you know why you struggle with some activities and do well in others. These tests are also available for you online.

Self-exploration

It will help you to better understand your own character traits. To do this, you may consider asking yourself questions like how you would describe yourself in a sentence, your purpose in life, how the most important thing that happened in your life changed you, or how different are you from those around you. Write it down in a sort of journal so you can check it anytime later.

Examine your strengths and weaknesses

Make a list of them and then compare what you discover with what the tests and your friends, family, or even co-workers say about you. Some strengths may include, determination, communication skills, creativity, empathy, imagination, adaptability among others. Weaknesses may be judgmental, self-centered, controlling, insecure, doubtful among others.

Know your day to day priorities

Ask yourself a question like if your house was on fire, what you would save? In which order? Whatever answer you come up with will determine your priorities. Family, Comfort, money, relationships, sex, security. You don't have to have the same priorities as others, but compare them to those around you that you hold in high esteem and you will tell a lot about you and the others. Knowing your priorities is a great step to start.

Look how you changed

Who you are is highly influenced by your past. Examine your past and think through what has happened to you over the years and how it has affected how you reason and behave today. Go back to when you were a child; what did you like to do then? What dreams did you have? What were you scared of? Love the little child you were because that child holds lots of answers you are looking for.

HOW TO DECLUTTER YOURSELF

In order to clear your path to self-discovery, the first thing to do is to declutter your life; your relationships, your home but also your thoughts. The things we keep with us physically and mentally impact directly our life, be it family, business wise or socially. Clutter in our physical surroundings and our relationships stops the flow of abundance and blocks happiness. When you have unwanted things in your life, that's clutter. There are certain things that you already know are clutter but there may be other useless things in your life that you do not know to carry. Well, all this clutter is leaving you with no space for the life you are longing for because is weighing you down like a stone tied to your foot. You wish to make things different but you keep lots of useless and old stuff taking your mind and space. This cluttering applies to your material, mental and emotional environment. Many times you hold on old relationships and experiences full of hate and refuse forgiveness. You have to be careful of those feelings because although they may make you feel rightful and powerful in your resentment, in reality they are just procrastinating you and stopping yourself to move forward.

Imagine that you are carrying a heavy load, won't it be better to get rid of the load and walk lighter? Holding on to the past will make difficult to be grateful and appreciative of the things in your life that matter. You must empty yourself in order to make space to build the new, you, your real you.

If you truly want a better version of you, do not procrastinate and make some changes in yourself and your habits. Start by getting rid of what is stopping you. Here are a few ways you can use to start decluttering yourself:

Your physical environment

Decluttering your physical environment is extremely important if you want to have a clear mind and attract abundance. This is the physical space you are in on daily basis — your home, place of work, and also your car. Eliminate those things that you no longer have the use for, as well as those things you don't need in your next phase of life. It is easier than you think and after doing it you will feel lighter and more free. Clean the space and keep it that way and you will notice the change that it does to your peace of mind. Even if you do not perceive it, the mind, unconsciously notices the surroundings all the time. There will be things that can go directly to the rubbish but others that can be given away because if they are not of use to you anymore they can be useful for other people. You may make others happy and help the planet too. Those things will keep on having their own use for another person who needs them after having served you, so you are not throwing anything just sharing with others. You can give them to charity or even sell them.

To start decluttering, try to visualize what you want for yourself in the future, how you want abundance and success in your life, where you desire to be in your next phase of life. Do you truly need the things you have in your vision? Do you have feelings and thoughts attached to things? Go through every room, drawers, and cabinets and evaluate if the things you have there are necessary for you. Do not hold to the past, but if you have objects that are emotional to you, just keep one of them as representation of the rest. Declutter everything, even things like the expired spices you have and have never used, mismatched socks, clothes that no longer fit, or even shoes that you don't wear anymore, furniture, toys, etc. This also includes those jeans two sizes smaller than yours that you keep in case you lose weight. It's time to let them go too. New goals can not be based in the past. You can wish to wear something for next season even keep a special dress, but not a few years old jeans. Think that once you have decluttered these items, you have created space for improved things and new items. If you declutter you will start gaining control of your life. Clear your space of the unwanted and unnecessary and become more organized to create harmony in your surroundings. This balance helps you keep a quieter mind and calls for new abundance in your life.

Your relationships

Healthy relationships enable us to be who we are, they nurture us and they help us grow. But relationships are challenging. They are a source of joy and comfort, but they can also bring a lot of pain. Relationships can cause us disappointment and let you feeling upset and hurt. You need to minimize your interactions with those who bring negativity into your life because they can even affect your health. Suppressing your feelings is unhealthy, especially when those feelings are anger or resentment.

Your life is influenced by those that you surround yourself with just like the physical stuff around you does. It is important to declutter your relationships because negative influences are likely to affect your life. Start with the people who put you down, the ones that criticize you but do not help you, the ones that do not care about you, and all those people that make you feel worthless. This doesn't mean that you won't see them again, but for now keep some distance and see how you feel. Do not blame them, just take some space from them and know that they too may have their own problems and are uncontrolled, but that they pouring them on to you knowingly or unknowingly. Do it as well with the 'bad influences' for instance, if you have friends that love partying all the time and you are always around them, of course, you will be partying too instead of doing or starting other things. You do not need to stop it suddenly, just reduce your party and drinking time. It is hard to make the change but, at a certain point, going out and partying becomes a habit and nearly an obligation and you become detached from life and unproductive. Think what your dreams and priorities really are. Who are those people, what are they bringing to your life and what is their future? Are you improving your life? Do you need to spend all your money in clothes to feel accepted by others? Do you really need new sneakers to make you happy?

The human mind is extremely receptive to suggestions especially if the suggestions were said by people we trust. People affect your life by setting their own expectations for your performance, worthiness and competence using labels such as "winner", "ugly", "fat", "boring" "loser", etc. You can become imprisoned by the labels they assign to you specially if you lack self-confidence because you may start believing them. The key to break free from the influence of others and to become confident and the first step to do so, is to know yourself and what you really want to accomplish in live. Otherwise you will live the live others want you to live, and so, get their approbation. But if that is not really what you want, you will still become very unhappy. Learn to know and love yourself and ignore their expectations, overlook the terms they use to describe you and instead focus on proving to them that they were wrong. Prove them true instead of trying to show others who they are. The easy part is proving those people wrong but the part that requires some effort is knowing yourself, accepting yourself, and finding your self-worth. In this book I will show you some tricks to do it. Don't let anybody determine your importance, worthiness or capabilities, instead show them who you are and focus on your goals. Self-confidence is all about not being obsessed with your weaknesses when you are around people. One of the key factors in feeling good about one's self is learning how to stop looking at your own flaws and weak points on constant basis when interacting with people. You need to stop to think of yourself negatively and accept yourself. **Self-**acceptance happens when you start changing your habits, life style and actions so that you find yourself worthy of being accepted. But you must persuade your subconscious mind to accept who you are. Suppose that you are shy and that is the reason you can't accept yourself. In such a case you should fight to develop social skills, read all articles about shyness and force yourself to deal with people. You will see that is not so difficult to interact with other people and you will start feeling more comfortable with others. Only then your subconscious mind will help you accept yourself because it will believe in you. Self-acceptance is not a passive action, it is about taking actions to remove the things and the factors that are preventing you from accepting yourself rather than staying defeated and trying to convince yourself that you love yourself.

Our self-esteem is never the same around everyone but it changes according to the people we are interacting with. You feel confident surrounded with your friends with no positive or negative thoughts in your mind but your self-esteem may differ according to the people you interact with. People usually feel less confident dealing with people who are successful, beautiful, powerful even certain family members. But think that this beautiful, successful or popular persons have their own fears, worries, problems and flaws. The main reason you feel so is that you compared yourself with one aspect of those person's personality to your personality, but you missed all the others aspects. Stop comparing yourself to others because you do not know all the facts. Instead focus on your goals and you may become like them.

For the time being, while you are trying to make a change, it will be helpful to take some distance or cut down these relations, even if they are family members. Take some time off to be with yourself and learn from yourself. Explore your relations, and be honest with yourself. Cut the cords and leave the relations that do you no good and are holding you down. This is the only way to improve and I assure you, once you start doing it you will realize how strong you are and see other possibilities you have in life. I bet you already know which relations affect you in a negative way but need to understand why. Now is your time, now is only you that matters. If you seek approval and acceptance from the others, you will always depend on someone else to feel completed and this is a direct sentence for unhappiness. You will never be able to please everyone, looks how successful people also have detractors, and know that people may change their mentality too. Your happiness starts with you and depends only on you: know yourself, accept yourself and love yourself because you are unique.

Emotional baggage

We all have a past full of experiences that with carry with us. This past needs to be explored and understood because it has built us in the way we are now. I will talk about it in a special chapter but for now understand how important it is to accept and make peace with what happened to you, your actions and reactions, and what you experienced in the past. Once you have done this work, you will learn forgiveness, which is the clue to liberation. If you don't forgive, the load of those feelings and emotions will keep burdening your spirit. If you start practicing forgiveness to self and others and you will get rid of revenge, regrets and shame. Don't hold on to bitterness because you will become a bitter person without knowing why, and you will keep on hurting and hindering yourself from moving forward emotionally. Do not allow fear, doubt and insecurity in your head. You need to get rid of the illusion of fear, it confuses you and confides you not to take risks or chances in life, thus gets in the way of your success. You have to allow yourself to heal. In life, things and situations will hurt and disappoint you, but do not hold on to the feelings of hurt and disappointment. Look at them as lessons learned and use them as stepping stones into your next level in life. If you want to live in your present and not in your past, release your frustrations. Decluttering your emotional baggage will help you see and recognize opportunities that come your way and take them.

Stress is also a big issue nowadays and it is also weighing you down. Avoid it by learning how to prioritize. Do not try to do everything at the same time, and start to do things or tasks according to their priority. Learn to accept you cannot do it all and delegate on others to free yourself. Do not be free to delegate; let go and free your time and mind.

These are the three areas where your life is usually cluttered. Only by decluttering them you will get a sense of freedom, self-worth, peace and control that will enable you to pursue the things you love and add value to your life.

BENEFITS OF DECLUTTERING

You will realize why it is so important to declutter your life by understanding its benefits. Anything that you do not use, like, or need is clutter and is holding you down. In the Feng-Shui philosophy, in order to create health, love, wealth, and overall abundance, you need free-flowing energy. Clutter hinders the energy flow and generates stagnation, exasperation, and exhaustion. Stagnant energy in your home is compared to rolling a boulder on top of a hill and letting it roll back on you anytime you rest. Everything you do needs of the life force and only by liberating yourself from the useless, you are able to create a new space and open streams of energy that will positively impact your life. Clutter in your life reflects the unfinished business that you may have. The following are some of the benefits you will experience once you start freeing yourself from impediments and arranging your mess:

You gain extra time

Once you declutter, you will notice that you have gained more time to do things that you love and you become more productive. You won't feel overwhelmed by the clutter in your home or workspace, and you find that you have more quality time for yourself and work more efficiently. For example: if you have a cluttered wardrobe, you spend a lot of time trying to find an outfit to wear when this time could be spend doing something else more fun or productive. When you declutter, you make your life easier for yourself, and more practical. You would be surprised to find yourself having an extra hour or two in a day after decluttering your space.

You feel lighter

After creating order and harmony in your home, you will feel more present and radiant. When you find yourself in spaces that are filled with fresh energy, inspiration and peace come in allowing magnetic areas of your personality become alive. The circulation of life energy force is the key to a vibrant life of health and abundance and it needs space to flow. Decluttering releases blockages and body imbalances to allow increased dynamism and wellness. Out with the old!

You can to do other things

When you get rid of blocks and unfinished business, new opportunities arise because you have more time and your mindset is open to new things. By clearing your life, you allow yourself to take bigger and more creative steps because the past is not holding you captive.

You start being able to address personal issues

As your workspace, your home and your wardrobe, you have to declutter your mind. This is the most important part of the decluttering because everything starts in your mind. When you cut through the mess in your daily life, it is possible to dig out some deep emotional clutter that has been buried. Everything including unpleasant memories or unachieved dreams have to be discovered and acknowledged. You need to do deep clean and you will realize that once you confront each unpleasant emotional clutter, you create room for a better and true you.

Helps you to discard your bad habits and start new ones

If you want to change your life you will have to start changing your habits, especially the bad ones. You already know which the most problematic are, but you may overlook others. In the book "The Power of Habit" by Charles Duhigg, he recommends to take a vacation as a way to break bad habits, because being outside of your comfortable habitat will help you to get free of the cues that trigger those bad habits. However, not everyone can afford a vacation away from home but you can always take a weekend or a short break to change things and create a new environment in your home. Clean the house, change the layout of the furniture and most important remove all the clutter that triggers the habits you have to give up on actions. For instance, if you need to be free of sugar, clear your pantry of sugar to avoid the habit of sugar binge and substitute it for healthier options, like fruits or nuts. By doing this, you remove triggers of negative emotions creating space for new positive habits and energy.

Better sleep

Clutter affects your subconscious mind and creates negative vibration, even if you do not perceive consciously and can cause you insomnia. The lack of sleep affects your mind and makes you unhealthy and the body needs to follow sleeping patterns. Experts recommend on average seven to eight hours of sleep to wake up rested and energized.

You learn how to keep focus

A fresh perspective that comes as a result of cleared mind and spaces give you the energy to solve other problems or any challenges. You are able to face your life more diligently because with free-flowing energy, your mind is able to objectively analyze the problems and find solutions faster.

You find yourself with more money

Decluttering your life, you stop buying unnecessary things and become more intentional about your spending. You begin to invest your money on things that are valuable instead of spending it carelessly. You may have debts like student loans or others that are causing you to be stressed and anxious, it might be because it has been increasingly difficult to service them. Decluttering helps you organize yourself financially and channel your money to more important goals, and even save money.

You gain trust in yourself

Clearing your space creates a sense of clarity and certainty and will you the feeling of having achieved something, at least a good start. You will gain more trust in the decisions you make because you will feel better.

As you see there are no disadvantages to decluttering your life, your mind and your space. When you declutter, you feel lighter, emotionally free, more energetic, and more dynamic. Life becomes easier, less stressful and more abundant. So go on, take that challenge to better yourself. Start slowly and with every step you make, feel the difference it brings to your life. Don't be afraid to take a chance. The first step is the hardest, but once you begin, your journey to freedom and happiness full of abundance is finally clear and can start.

DECLUTTERING YOUR MIND

Many people when they hear about decluttering, they think only about their physical environment but forget that the way we think is determining our life. It is worse to have a cluttered mind than a cluttered home. When your mind is cluttered, it is unfocused and restless. Your mind tends to wander in different directions and preventing you from your personal goals because there is little that you get done.

Some of the things that clutter your mind include worrying about the future, being stuck in your past, having a to-do list in the mind, complaining, insecurity and ungratefulness. Thankfully, there are numerous strategies that will help you to clean out some clutter in your mind.

Decluttering your physical environment

Mental clutter can be as a result of physical clutter. Clutter crowds the mind with unnecessary stimuli that force the brain to work on overload. Physical clutter communicates to the brain that there is so much more to get done which is exhausting to the mind. When you declutter your physical environment, you soon discover your mind feels freer and you can think more clearly.

Note it down

Don't try to remember everything; it is impossible and stresses the brain because of the amount of information we need to use in our daily life and the fear of failing. Choose an easier tool by practicing to note down your to-do list, passwords, appointments, and so forth. You can choose a digital way like noting on your phone or laptop or even putting it down on paper. Think of it as your storage device for those bits of information that you require to remember. It will also help you to have an overview of what needs to be done and help you to organize yourself accordingly.

Journal keeping

Keeping a journal is more detailed than noting down. A journal allows you to write your inner thoughts, not just what you want to do. It helps you evaluate yourself and understand the things that may be clogging your mind. You may write about things you worry about, your plans for achieving certain goals in life, any concerns you may be having, maybe about a relationship or your work, your night dreams and your goals. A journal helps you to understand yourself and focus on your life.

Let go of your past

Past can really drag you down. Many people are not able to move forward because of the clutter of the past stored at the back of their minds. They cloud their minds with past mistakes, missed opportunities, past hurt aches, and grievances. It is important that you take your time, go through your mental closets, and get rid of memories of the past that serve no purpose in your current life. In this book you will find the ways to release your mind from your painful past and clear space for pleasant present memories.

Try not to multitask

Avoid doing multiple tasks at the same time. Research shows that those that multi-task are less productive than those that focus on one task at a time. Multitasking strains your mind. Instead of multitasking, try prioritizing your tasks, pick what is most important and essential, and tackle each task as the need arises. Practice delegating. Do not try to do more than you are able to do but do what you are sure and able to do.

Filter the information coming in

Don't allow too much information to come your way. A lot of information clogs your brain and causes confusion. Information come from blogs, television and social media among other areas. Create space by practicing the following tips:

- Put a limit on time spent on social media and browsing the internet.
- Look at your magazine subscriptions and cancel those that don't add value to your life. Unsubscribe from unnecessary blogs in your life and create space for more valuable ones.
- Ensure that the opinions you pick are from credible individuals.
- Chose information that is relevant to you and cut off all others.

Be decisive

Do not procrastinate on decision making. If you keep postponing the decisions to make, soon your brain will be clogged with decisions that need to be made and must be made. The solution, be decisive. Create a list of pros and cons to help you make a decision about a certain thing. Only by being decisive can you change your life, the way you feel now and put you in the right path to attain your goals.

Autopilot routine decisions

Small routine decisions that may seem easy can take a lot of time and occupy a lot of brain space. These may include decisions on breakfast each morning, clothes to wear, or even what to have for lunch. To help with this, you can have a meal timetable for each week. Schedule the time and day to do certain tasks like laundry. Assign a day that you go out to meet your friends and so forth. If you realize, people like Steve Jobs or Mark Zuckerberg always wear the same outfit, as if it was their personal uniform. So do politicians, most of bank people, lawyers because in this way they do not need to worry about what to wear every day and they invest this time in something else instead. Try to find your work uniform adding little changes and you will simplify your life.

Prioritize

When you find you have an endless list of things to do, you will get exhausted even before you begin doing any. Accept that you can't do all because the day has only 24 hours. Prioritize by choosing and focusing on the most important tasks to you. List your priorities and focus on them.

Learn meditation

Meditation is learning to have your mind focused on the now and stop it from wandering. In the following chapters, you will learn how to mediate putting all your attention on one thing at a time, like breathing and you will notice how all other thoughts disappear. Meditate will help you to make the useless and unnecessary thoughts disappear from your mind.

When your mind is cluttered, so is your brain, leading to a congested inner world. This state of mind blocks your ability to think clearly and to focus on the things that are important. Try and practice the above 10 simple tips to empty and declutter your mind for a true, healthier and happier you.

YOUR EGO CAN WORK AGAINST YOU

What is ego? Ego is defined as the conscious mind of a person, that part that one considers to be the 'self' and different to the rest. For instance, when you say a person has a big ego, it simply means that they are full of themselves. Ego according to the Cambridge Dictionary is also defined as the idea you have of yourself, your feelings of how important you are and your abilities in the world. Another definition of Ego according to Sigmund Freud, ego is a part of the personality that internalizes the requirements of the superego, and reality. The basic part of your personality that encourages people to fulfill their primary needs is the id. The moralistic part of your personality that forms from your childhood and influenced by your socialization is what is called the superego. The work of the ego, therefore, is to create a balance between the id and superego by making sure the needs of the id are met and confirmation of the superego to reality.

Ego can be your friend or your foe, the choice is yours. However, it is important to note that you cannot get rid of your ego as long as you have your physical body. It is important to have an ego just as it is important to have a mind and intellect. Since you cannot get rid of your ego, your best choice is to balance it and ensure it is in harmony with the rest of your life. In your earlier life, the ego is dormant, but from the age of 2, you start discovering about self in simple things like ownership and identifying what belongs to you. This discovery may be challenging to those around you, but this is the time you enter into a period where ego plays a very important role in your life. As you grow, you realize the ego is necessary for establishing your life, it helps you in your education, career, having a family among other things. The ego is controlling the things around you and your life, as well as organizing it, that is why is so important to have a healthy Ego.

Taken to the extreme, a person can become egocentric. An egocentric is someone who is limited in outlook or concern to his or her own activities or needs concerned with the individual rather than society. It means thinking only of oneself, without regard for the feelings or desires of others; self-centered and self-absorbed. Note that on an egocentric person is also the one who feels responsible for everything bad or good that happens. When not managed, the negative aspect of ego can manifest into arrogance, judgments, vanity, prejudices, and even pride. In some extreme cases, it manifests itself as the need to be controlling, lustful for power, fanaticism, and an obsession of material things. This is the period where the ego can be troublesome because it makes the personal delusional and detached from the real life. The ego starts controlling you while conflicting with your spiritual side that wants to break the boundaries and live in freedom. When you engage in your spiritual practice, often your ego comes in between because it does not want to change. It will try to procrastinate your will by having thoughts such as: 'you tried a diet last month and it didn't work, neither will this new spiritual journey'. However, if you stop listening to your mind and continue with your spiritual journey, the ego will start to panic by realizing change is inevitable. The first step is not to listen to the mind but put all your energy on the goals that will improve yourself and your life.

The fuel for ego is fear. The ego does not like changes and will try to keep the things as they are. If allowed, ego will put fear into all areas of your life and paralyze you from moving forward. It will use negative traits such as insecurity, lack of self-worth, lust, greed, anger, or intolerance, all rooted in fear with the ego. Your ego understands all your weaknesses, repressed desires, and denials, and will use them against you and try to make you to fall off your journey. It will create self-doubt and worries and make you start questioning what you are doing, if you are on the right track, whether the new You is going to bring you real happiness and so forth.

When these thoughts come your way, you need to counter them by asking yourself if this is your ego or your higher self. You have to learn to control it instead of letting the ego control you. As long as you live, your ego will be with you but it is of absolute importance to remain focused and vigilant about your ego and instill self-discipline too.

To successfully manage your ego, you must live your life intentionally and consciously. You must be aware of the choices you make, why you make them, and their impact on yourself and those around you. Also, it is important to watch your words by asking yourself questions like "Is it true?", "Is it kind?" or "is it necessary?" Set your goals in front of your ego and be disciplined in what you want to achieve in life. All said and done, love your ego and learn how to play with and manage it to your own good You do not have to get rid of it, what you need to is to have a balanced ego that works in your favor instead of against you. Meditation will help you to understand your ego and manage it more successfully because you will be taking time to sit with yourself and know yourself better. One of the most important things in your life is to understand your ego and how it works, so you can learn how to make it positive and useful for you because the ego is one, if not the most, powerful of your weapons. It is your idea of your self-esteem, self-importance, self-worth, self-respect, self-conceit, self-image, self-confidence, and if it is not balanced or in accordance with the reality, it will play tricks on you.

Your ego can stand in your way of growth. As earlier discussed, ego can be founded on false confidence or false insecurity both fueled by fear and ignorance of the self. Ego can work against you if you are not careful and allow it to rule your life. There are four things that you need to understand about ego:

Projection of the wrong image – When you allow an unbalanced ego to control you, you are likely to portray the wrong image to those around you. You are easily misunderstood because you allow the wrong image of who you truly are to be seen, plus you are unable to recognize the others as they really are.

Know that ego is not your true self – Ego can boost you with false confidence or false insecurity. If you are not careful, your ego will create obstacles into your growth because you also begin to believe what the ego is projecting.

Never take your ego seriously – Your ego can create obstacles in your relationship with others because of the insecurities, overconfidence, or even delusion that separate you from your true self and the real life.

Be honest about yourself – be confident of who you are, your strengths, and weaknesses. When you are honest, you automatically take away the power of your ego and hence you grow bigger than your ego.

Signs that your ego is in control

Do you feel responsible for everything that happens? Have you ever found yourself doing or saying something that causes you to cringe? Have you felt embarrassed and ashamed about your reactions without understanding why you had them? Are you sometimes surprised about your behavior? Do you hate that sense of insecurity? Are you having problems controlling your anger? Do you have the need to always win and when you lose you feel devastated? If so, it is very likely that the culprit is your ego. It is not easy to manage your ego and if you are not careful and very watchful, you will find yourself doing uncontrolled things that are not beneficial to you. In simple terms, the ego has been defined as that part of us that makes us feel the need to be more special and it will always try to be different and separated to everything and everyone else. Remember that the Ego is the part of the mind that mediates between the conscious and the unconscious and it is responsible for reality testing and a sense of personal identity.

The ego is not about arrogance or being overly confident, it is about feeling more worthy and superior or worthless and inferior to others without it being real. Sometimes, you may look at yourself and feel that you are not good enough or even compare yourself to others and feel like you are not good enough. This is your ego causing you an inferiority complex.

In order to control your ego, you must be aware of it. You must master how to recognize when your ego is at play and control it before it is too late. For that you will need to make a self-check in an objective way, which is quite difficult as the ego will interfere. There are a few signs that will help you notice if your ego is taking control, these are:

1. You feel energized after talking about other people's weaknesses or failures.
2. You find yourself in a heated argument and the only way you back down is if you win it.
3. You find yourself constantly comparing yourself with others and seeing yourself not good enough, desiring to be like them.
4. You constantly look down on people. You look at other people and feel they are not as good as you.

5. You are jealous of other people's accomplishments.

6. You focus on self, talk about yourself so much more before even asking others how they are.

7. You prefer winning to doing your best.

8. You are a sour loser. You believe in winning all the time and sulk when you don't.

9. You set unattainable goals for yourself and beat yourself up if you don't attain them.

10. You never accept responsibility. You blame others when things go wrong or not your way.

Ways in which the ego works against you

Remember earlier, we talked how the ego likes being in control and in regard to decluttering yourself to live better, you will have to understand your own ego and learn to control it. A step to decluttering yourself means that you are taking charge over your life and your ego may not like it and will work against sabotaging the new you. There are a few characteristics of the ego that will work against you, these include:

Ego hates change.

This is one of the greatest fears of ego. The ego loves comfort and status quo and does not appreciate the change. An egocentric person sees fault in others and prefers they change but not him. Decluttering your mind is a change that your ego will fight you on and you will even begin to have doubts in the process.

Ego will trivialize the clutter of the mind and focus on the physical clutter.

Earlier, it was discussed that the worst clutter you can have it is that of the mind. Your ego is formed through external forces like the need for validation, jobs, opinions, or education. It will focus on eliminating what it considers to be external sings that are measurable. Ego can allow you to declutter your physical environment but hold you back from decluttering your nonphysical environment thus the mind by instilling fear of the change.

Ego needs to be considered special and reluctantly acknowledges others.
Your ego is selfish. It focuses on you and what pleases you and refuses to acknowledge others. Your ego, if not controlled, will steal the spotlight and most often will manipulate others to achieve attention. It resents anyone that would threaten its reputation.

Your ego holds on to the past, dreams of the future but refuses to live in the present
The ego usually has an unhealthy attachment to your past and the future. It makes you think of 'the good old days', or falsely manipulate you into thinking how things used to be in the past, holding you captive in your past and refusing you to move forward. The ego believes in restoring the old way of doing things to solve problems and is very scared of the future because it is unknown.

The ego loves quick gratification and hates hard things.
If it needs effort, it is hard or causes you discomfort, your ego tells you it is not worth pursuing. Instead of struggling with uncomfortable situations or anxiety, your ego will go out for quick solutions. Decluttering your life is not easy, it is physically and mentally draining and your ego is likely to discourage you and cause you to give up and look for a quick fix.

The ego is sensitive and easily takes offense.
Do you easily feel offended? When the ego is in control, nearly every disagreement or differing point of view feels like a targeted attack. To counter this, the ego seeks to be around people of like-mindedness in order to gain validation. As you embark on the journey of decluttering yourself, it is most likely that you will be corrected or told the way that you were doing things before is wrong and how you should do things from now. Your ego

will not be happy with this and will start seeking for others that are not changing their lives and manipulate you as to why you should not change. After all, your friends are happy, yet they are not changing.

If you don't take control of your ego and allow for balance, you are likely to find discouragement from within yourself. The little voice in your mind will start to judge and criticize you. It is not easy to manage your ego, but with the above understanding, you are likely to recognize when the ego is taking control over you and control it. Your ego can stand in your way of progress by posing very convincing arguments in your mind. Learn how to know if it is your ego speaking to you or is it your higher self. Don't let it be the gap in your life.

The Mirror Meditation

Exercise: The spiritual teacher Osho taught a technique for mirror meditation in Dynamics of Meditation. His method encouraged a private practice in a darkened room, a candle by the side of the mirror by which one sat. That mirror gazing is a very strong technique to your own abyss look and get acquainted with your own naked reality. This exercise will also help you to stop identifying yourself with your mind. He suggested practicing it during sixty days in a 40 minutes session in which the practitioner simply stared into his or her own eyes trying not to blink. My advice is that you to start with 10-15 minutes and add five more minutes every three days. Try to write down what you see and feel so you can reread it later.

Mirror meditation works like this: before you go to bed stand alone in front of a mirror, if it is large the better. You should be in a dark space lighted only by a candle. Your face should be in the mirror, not the flame. Now stare into your own eyes in the mirror and try not to blink. If you do, go back to stare in your eyes. Even if tears are welling up, let them come, but try not blinking and keep staring at your eyes. At some point you will notice something very peculiar: the face in the mirror takes other forms. The face in the mirror begins to change and reveal the many faces of ourselves. It can be disconcerting at first, because these essences that appear are very real and often quite unfamiliar, from other places, worlds and times. But they are merely aspects of the self. Your unconscious mind begins to explode. Then one day, something extremely strange happens: suddenly you see no face in the mirror. You stare into the void, that is the moment! Then close your eyes and encounter the unknown.

UNDERSTANDING YOUR MIND

BUDDHIST KNOWLEDGE OF THE MIND

I have a question for you: Do your thoughts have control over you or do you have control over your thoughts? Your mind belongs to you, and you have authority over what you think and say and believe. Just because a thought comes into your head doesn't mean it's yours; it doesn't mean you have to think about it or entertain it. In this book you will learn how to do it. The first two chapters are more theoretical because you need to comprehend how the mind works and how your uncontrolled thoughts are affecting your life.

As you seek to understand your mind, it is important to know what your mind is. The mind is not the brain. The brain is a physical part of your body that you can see, can be operated on, or even photographed. The mind, on the other side, has a non-physical nature of the mind. It has been defined as a continuum that is formless and works by perceiving and understanding objects. Because of t, physical objects cannot obstruct it.

The Buddhist teach that *everything is fundamentally dependent upon the mind*. Our worldly experiences are as a result of karma (our actions), and all our actions originate from the mind. To change your world, one must begin by changing their mind. This can only be achieved by your understanding of how the mind works. This book will provide you with detailed explanations of the types of minds and its reactions and it offers you practical advice on how you can improve your life. By understanding your mind, you will be taking the first steps to your final liberation.

It is important to differentiate the two states of mind: the disturbed and the peaceful one. The main causes of our suffering are the state of minds that disturb our peace. These states are those of jealousy, anger, and delusion. Suffering does not come from other people but from our own disturbed state of mind. Learn to be responsible for your thoughts. According to Buddhist teaching, permanent liberation from suffering can only be achieved by purifying the mind. If you desire to be free from problems and gain eternal peace and happiness, you must improve your understanding of your own mind and the knowledge behind it.

In this book I am going to talk about meditation, because it creates peace of the mind and that is what you need to live the life the way you one. When you free your mind from distractions, the opinion of others, and thought talking, it becomes open, peaceful and calm. Your internal peace will make you regain content. Your body and mind become easy, comfortable. One of the benefits of certain practices like concentration is the flexibility of the mind, the rate at which the mind can be serviced. When you meditate, you get a certain small level of suppleness, you gain adaptability in mental actions but with more practice on concentration, you get stronger and stable. It is important for the mind suppleness to be long-lasting because so it won't make you get mentally or physically tired. At the beginning it seems impossible to mediate for fifteen or even for five minutes, but with practice you will be able to last in meditation for much longer periods.

Your worst enemy is laziness which is not about sleep only or physical ease, but it means that the mind has declined to engage in what beneficial for you. The mind is controlling your willpower. That is why it is very important to eliminate this laziness and stop the mind when it starts having this can of thoughts. Do not listen to it, instead, engage, for example, in meditation, painting, sport or reading, something that will keep your mind busy. Anything you may decide to do will be beneficial for you, even go out for a walk. You just need a little start and you will see how ignoring the voice of your mind becomes easier. For example, if you had an appointment at the gym and start think about the weather to make an excuse, just do not listen, go out to the gym and after your training notice how you feel and ask yourself why was your mind trying to sabotage you. Try to do anything that it is good for you and will distract your mind. The Americans have a say: *"If today I do something that you don't do, tomorrow I will do something that you can't do"*. Excuses won't take you near to your goals and dreams, excuses will paradise you and keep you stuck. Do not listen to the excuses it will use to procrastinate you, follow your goals and ignore it; remember it is scared of change and will fight to leave its comfort zone.

Concentration is important too. When you lack concentration, your mind is uncontrolled and as a result, it can easy fall into sadness, anger, hatred, attachment, or any other delusion. With concentration, you can tame it to do what you want and become in control of your mind. To fully understand your mind, concentration is key not only during meditation but also to stop the negative thoughts and help you to achieve your goals. By developing concentration skills, with meditation and focus, you will find peace of mind and also empower your mind abilities. You have the power to change your mind. Accept that you cannot change other people or the circumstances you find yourself in, because illness, suffering and death are part of life and they are unavoidable. What makes the real difference is how you react, how your mind is trained to face the problems, changes and the unexpected events that will occur during your life.

THE MONKEY MIND

The term *Monkey Mind* according to the Buddhist principles refers to being restless, unsettled, or confused, a mind that jumps from one idea to another, like a monkey from tree to tree. The *Monkey Mind* is also referred to as the inner critic and it is said to be that part connected to your ego. This is the part that claims you cannot do anything right. It is also the part that blocks your creativity and hinders you from progressing forward with the things that you love. This unsettled mind always insists that it must be heard and it requires a lot of self-control to silence it. It is also where you find yourself easily distracted and if you need to get something done in your life, your biggest challenge is to silence the Monkey Mind.

In order to silence your mind, the first step would be to become calm and firm. Try to focus on being present, being in the here and now, being in the moment in other words, become mindful. I am sure you have already heard these terms from the Mindfulness trend, but it has been known for centuries, that when you are mindful, you embrace awareness and interconnection between your inner world and outer world. This is important, because when you are more alert, you realize that you are really alive. You become aware of yourself and your place in the world. Stop walking like in a dream you do not understand and start paying attention to the thoughts that cross your mind, your body and your surroundings, and you will notice all the difference.

Buddha explained the human mind using the metaphor that it is full of drunk monkeys chattering and jumping from one tree branch to the next without stopping. This means that your mind is in constant motion. The chatter of your thoughts could be like:

- Your mind is thinking about your laundry and a to-do list.
- Your mind is focusing on real and imagined fears.
- Your mind is thinking of your past and the pain.
- Your mind is criticizing your present.
- Your mind is worrying and creating fears of the future.

A *Monkey Mind* makes it impossible for you to enjoy the present because you cannot slow down. There is also a lot of negativity with your mind affecting your mood causing you to be angry, unhappy, anxious, and restless. Your ability to concentrate is hampered with and often has a negative impact on your behavior, as well as the ability to positively interact with others. Having dozens of monkeys in your brain is also very stressful and puts a barrier to our day to day lives. However, there is good news. It is possible to get your *Monkey Mind* to calm down.

You need to tame your thoughts to increase your clarity of the mind, gain sense of well-being and calmness, improve the concentration in what you do, even sleep better, but you need to do it specially to gain control of your life and set your goals.

How to tame your Monkey Mind

It is possible to tame your Monkey Mind but you have to know how and practice. Up till now you have let your Monkey Mind to keep running wild, meaning that your thoughts run through your mind without control. Don't allow your thoughts to rule you but rule your thoughts.

Talk to your Monkey Mind

It is possible to have a conversation with your *Monkey Mind*. When it is fully up, have a conversation to calm it down. Listen to what it is saying, understand why it is upset, and why all the chatter, then do this:

- If it is trying to remind you of something that needs your attention or to be done, make a note of it and allocate the time to do it. This will calm your thoughts and will stop it from worrying about it.
- Do you have anxiety about the future? Talk to it and reassure it that all is well. Come up with a contingency plan together after conducting a worst-case scenario.
- Does your mind project hate or resentment over a past issue? It about time that you do something to deal with your past so that it is not brought up again by your *Monkey Mind*.

Sometimes the *Monkey Mind* wants to be listened too. Once it feels it has been heard and action is taken, it settles down.

Start a journaling practice

This is a deliberate effort to listen to your Monkey Mind. Establish a journaling practice that is regular by setting aside time each day to deal with your Monkey Mind's concerns. You do it by:

- Allowing your mind to run amok for a few minutes every day at a specific time. Let your Monkey Mind understand this.
- At this time, write down every feeling and thoughts that comes to you and your worries as well.
- Learn to stop after consuming the amount of time that you allocated to journaling.

Once you are done, communicate to your *Monkey Mind* that the time is up and that you will not give it any more attention until the following day during journaling. If your *Monkey Mind* starts some chatter later on in the day, refuse to give it any attention. By practicing this, your Monkey Mind will soon understand that it is worthless to create a raucous any other time other than the time for journaling.

Meditate

This is the most effective technique to calming your Monkey Mind. When you meditate, you train your mind to stay still as you regain power and control over it. With daily practice, you gain skill in keeping your monkey quiet and being able to silence the Monkey Mind at will.

Use the A-B-C technique

When your thoughts disagree with your surroundings, your *Monkey Mind* is activated. When your current moment does not agree with the demands of your Monkey Mind, it starts to chatter. To avoid this, practice the A-B-C technique as it will assist you to deal with the disparity between your *Monkey Mind* thoughts and actual happenings. How does this technique work?

- A is about 'activating event'. This is the current thing happening.
- B is for your beliefs. Your personal beliefs cause your monkey brain to start interpreting whatever is happening.

- C is about consequences. These are the results arrived at because of what is currently happening, that is feeling certain emotions.

The key to this technique is to question the beliefs that the *Monkey Mind* is basing its conclusions upon. Some examples of the questions you may ask are:

- Are people obliged to act the way you want them to act all the time?
- Must things always go your way and how realistic is that?
- Is it true that you must always perform well?

Should you reject the beliefs that your *Monkey Mind* relies upon to justify its temper, it will no longer bother you about the same and will calm down the thoughts on that issue.

Do not assign meaning

This simply means letting your senses take into your surroundings and then stop. Don't allow your *Monkey Mind* to jump and form a judgment, criticize, and assigns meaning. When you begin doing this regularly, you will discover that you start to see things clearer than before and as if that's not enough, you begin to see so much more than you did.

Recite a Mantra

When your *Monkey Mind* starts to chatter, you can interrupt and distract it by reciting a mantra. You can use *"Om mani padme hum"* but know that a mantra can be a word that you keep reciting like 'peace'. Reciting a mantra helps you to stop the flow of thoughts and bring in your scattered attention and be able to focus on a word. A mantra can be recited silently or audibly. When your goal is to tame your mind, recite it loudly. This enables you to listen to the word, sound, or phrase engaging your hearing senses. It is much easier to tame your thoughts if you are able to stimulate more senses. A mantra is usually a positive word or phrase. By repeating it silently or audibly, you find that you are listening to positive things as opposed to the negative being initiated by your *Monkey Mind.*

Engage in the game of fives
When you hear the first monkey chattering in your mind, that's when you realize your mind has wandered off from the present moment. This is the time to bring all the monkeys in your mind back to the present. A method that is used to bring the mind back is by engaging in the game of fives. Relax your thoughts and notice five things around you. They can be through sight, smell, or sound. This you do by pretending you have never encountered the smell, sound, or sight by adopting every sense in wonder. When you do this, your attention is drawn to the present and your Monkey Mind goes silent.

Involve your mind
Have you ever experienced a moment of your mind being totally still? That your experiences are of the current goings and not your mind chattering and giving you narration of events as they occurred? Your mind may go still when you are reading, watching a movie, or even writing—a moment of total concentration.
Engaging your mind is one of the most effective ways to silence your *Monkey Mind.* If you feel your *Monkey Mind* is driving you crazy, look for an activity that completely takes your attention, hence no room left to listen to your monkey thoughts.
Get creative and engage in painting, writing, reading or gardening. These activities will keep your mind busy and away from your stress focus. You will gain peace of mind and the rewards of a new art piece , a beautiful garden and Knowledge. This time investment in yourself will bring you rewards that will make a positive impact in you.

Practice Piko-Piko breathing
Piko means center or navel. This breathing technique is from the ancient philosophy of the Hawaiian Huna. The technique involves:

- Deeply breathing in. When inhaling, focus your attention to the crown of your head.
- As you exhale, focus your attention on your navel.
- Continue breathing, switching your attention between the crown of your head and your navel.
- Repeat several times

Breathing deeply while focusing your attention on a certain spot then automatically move to focus on another spot helps calm your *Monkey Mind*.

As you see there are many benefits of taming your *Monkey Mind*. It takes practice to be able to calm your thoughts, but the good news is that it can be done. The mind loves to play, like a monkey, so the best way to control it is by playing tricks on it The hints discussed above will greatly help you to tame your *Monkey Mind*. Start now and see yourself transforming to live your true and best life yet.

BUDDHA GAUTAMA

Now we are going to talk about Buddhism and how Buddha began his quest for enlightenment and underwent a transformation that set in place a spiritual revolution that is still practiced today. Note that his teaching shows a way of life that can be followed and practiced by any person regardless of their religious affiliations. His teachings are a guide to self-discipline of the body, mind and word, self-purification and development, and is not based on any beliefs, prayers, or ceremonies.

Siddhartha Gautama was born in Lumbini as the son of a king. The young prince was raised in a privileged life full of luxury and protected from the knowledge of pain and suffering. At the age of 29, he left his family to go interact with his subjects and this is when he came face to face with the reality of human suffering. The first four sights he saw were that of a sick person, an old person, a dead person, and a holy man. These sights greatly disturbed him to the point to renounce his life and go on a quest to understand the truth of birth and death in order to seek the peace of mind. He engaged in strict yoga practices and serious asceticism. He allowed torture upon his own body, yet he still did not find enlightenment. Then one day, he remembered something that had happened to him as a boy. He remembered sitting under a rose-apple tree and how he experienced a great bliss and entered a deep meditative state. He discovered that the way to realization did not mean punishing his body to find peace, but to work with his environment and find the purity of the mind. At point Buddha realized that the path to awakening was a balance between extremes of self-denial and self-indulgence of life. A young girl offered him rice and milk and he ate them, but when his ascetic companions, saw him eating, they thought that he had given up on his quest and abandoned him.

He went to the north of India and at Bodh Gaya, Gautama sat under a sacred fig tree and decide that he would sit and meditate until he would understand live. Once he had absorbed himself in meditation and purified his mind by concentration, he acquired the knowledge of his past lives and the past lives of all beings; the laws of karma; and how to be free from obstacles and release from attachments. But then he encountered a demon called Mara who tried to tempt him unsuccessfully. After defeating the demon Mara with its soldiers, Siddhartha Gautama discovered enlightenment and became a Buddha.

Buddha wanted to spread the knowledge he had gained for people to liberate themselves too, and started to teach the Four Noble Truths and the Eightfold Path.

The Four Noble Truths

The Noble Truths are the center of the Buddha's teaching. These are the four truths that he summarized his teachings on.

1. The first truth is that of suffering
2. The second truth is the origin of suffering
3. The third truth is of cessation of suffering

4.   The fourth truth is the path to the cessation of suffering

With the first two truths, he established the problem and identified its cause. The third truth speaks about a cure for the suffering or the problem, and the fourth truth is the medicine or the way to achieve the cure by setting out the Eightfold Path.

The First Noble Truth is Suffering - Dukkha

Life is suffering - There are many ways that suffering comes into our lives. The three obvious sufferings are associated with: old age, death, and sickness. However, according to Buddha, suffering is much deeper. Life is not always fair. Most often, it fails to meet your expectations. The nature of human beings is to have desires and cravings, but their satisfaction is short-lived because should it be experienced for long, it becomes boring and monotonous. You may suffer from external causes like sickness or bereavement, but the internal suffering of lack of satisfaction or fulfillment is the true suffering.

The human sufferings are: the suffering of birth, aging, sickness and death; the suffering of separation and being parted from what you like; the suffering of encountering what you dislike; not obtaining the object of your desire. To make up our identity we collectively use make the body, physical feelings, mental fabrications (thoughts and fantasies, feelings, images), and our perception and consciousness. But we forget the important fact that everything changes all the time and that life is constantly evolving and nothing lasts forever. Life is impermanent and this is why we cannot depend or rely on things, persons, places or other external factors and truly identify them as part of "me, mine or what I am" because this is how dis-satisfaction and suffering occurs in life.

You may think these Buddhist teachings are neither optimistic nor pessimistic. They are the reality and even if we try to avoid them, they are part of the life. But these teachings do not end with suffering, because Buddha also explained what to do and how to end the suffering.

The Second Noble Truth is The Origin of Suffering - Samudaya

The root of suffering is desire - In the second noble truth, the Buddha said to have found the true causes of suffering. You are likely to think that your pain and suffering is caused by obvious things like injury, sadness when you have lost someone or anything that you can identify with. The Buddha says that causes of suffering are much deeper than what we worry about on a daily basis. The cause of human suffering lies in ignorance of the reality and Karma. Ignorance and its resulting Karma have often times been called "desire" or craving in his teachings, he says that the single most cause of suffering is desire – Tanha. There are three forms of desire and cravings:

- Craving for sensual pleasures such as love, money, fame or power, pleasures or good health.
- Craving for further becoming is wanting our life to be so that things will continue, believe that you will live forever, that the good times will always stay.
- Craving for non-becoming finally is wanting for things to not happen, such as death, poverty, pain, illness or problems.
- These cravings come in what Buddhists call the "Three poisons":
- Desire and greed.
- Delusion or ignorance of the reality.
- Destructive desires or urges and hatred.

When you start wishing things were different and you attached yourself to ideas, promises and desires of how these things should be, but your mental and physical powers cannot make them be exactly what you want, then you are building foundation of all your unhappiness. Some of the root afflictions are:

- Desire, attached to internal or external objects
- Anger or hatred
- Pride: thinking oneself superior to other lower persons, fancying superior to those who are equal, thinking oneself slightly inferior to

other who in reality are superior.

- Ignorance which in this context is a non-realizing consciousness that obstructs one from seeing the actual reality.
- Wrong view of oneself over or underestimating the own qualities, identifying oneself with those qualities.
- Doubt about what to do.

The Third Noble Truth is The Cessation of Suffering - Nirodha

The third noble truth talks about the possibility of freedom or liberation. The Buddha lived life to show that it was possible to eliminate desire by relinquishing any attachments to things. He taught that to eliminate desire as a cause of suffering, you need to find freedom from attachment. The teachings further say that when a person finds the truth, they find Estrangement, meaning they are disenchanted, so they become aware of their surroundings and senses but are not swayed by them.

Think about the faults of attachment: the object never lasts because life is impermanent, plus your desire may change and it won't fulfill your grasping anymore; you may be exaggerating the importance of the object and this will lead to future disappointment; and meanwhile in your mind arise feelings of possessiveness, anger, jealousy, pride, fear and insecurity in case of loss.

>*"As long as you follow attachment,*
>*satisfaction is never found.*
>*Whoever reverses attachment*
>*with wisdom, attains satisfaction".*
>*Lord Buddha*

Nirvana in the Buddhist teachings means extinguishing. Through knowledge you can manage to extinguish or eliminate all the three poisons of delusion, hatred, and greed, and eventually attain Nirvana. When you reach nirvana, you have reached a state of mind that is of pure joy with no negative emotions and fears.

The Fourth Truth is The Cessation of Suffering - Magga

This is the final truth where Buddha gives a prescription on how to end suffering. This fourth truth is based on a set of 8 principles that he called the *'Eightfold Path'*. This is also called the Middle way where one obtains balance in life which lays in between indulgence and asceticism.

THE EIGHTFOLD PATH

The Eightfold path is a set of principles to help in the ending of suffering according to the Buddhist teachings. It is derived from the fourth noble truth and it is further grouped into 3 important parts of the Buddhist practice. The three elements are the moral conduct, wisdom, and mental discipline. The 8 principles or eightfold path consists of:

- Right understanding
- Right thought
- Right speech
- Right action
- Right livelihood
- Right effort
- Right mindfulness
- Right concentration

The whole teaching of the Buddha is based on the four truths and the end of suffering which can be found following the *Eightfold Way*. It is encouraged to develop the eight principles together, although it doesn't mean that you must develop them according to how they are listed. They are linked together with each principle being able to help the other, hence the need to try and develop them simultaneously.

The eight principles are further grouped into 3 elements of mental discipline, ethical conduct, and wisdom.

Ethical Conduct

According to Buddhism, in order for you to be perfect, you must develop two qualities: compassion and wisdom. Under compassion, you find charity, love, kindness, and tolerance, but you also need the wisdom of the mind. You cannot develop one quality and neglect the other. If you developed the qualities of emotions and forgot about wisdom, then you will be a compassionate person that is acting foolish because without knowledge you will be doing the wrong things, for example not helping others in the right way. The aim of Buddhist teaching, therefore, is for you to develop both equally. Under the ethical conduct, there are three principles of the eightfold path. These are the right action, speech, and livelihood.

Right Speech

Right speech means not telling lies, no gossiping or slander, or any talk that brings hatred, disunity, enmity, or disharmony among people, no harsh, impolite, abusive, malicious or rude language, no idle, useless, and stupid gossip. When you abstain from these wrongs, you will automatically speak the truth and be mindful of your language and how it impacts on others. Before you start talking think whether what you are going to say is true and necessary to be told, and do it with kindness.

Right Action

Advocates for honorable, peaceful, and moral conduct. You should abstain from destroying life, stealing, having illegitimate sexual pleasures, dishonest dealings, because all this actions will bring you suffering. Instead you should be of help to others.

Right Livelihood

This means that you should earn your living from a profession that does not cause harm to others.

These three factors (right actions, speech, and livelihood) constitute ethical conduct. The aim of the Buddhist ethical and moral conduct is to encourage a harmonious life at both a personal level and societal level.

Mental Discipline

Here, three more factors of the eightfold path are included. Right effort, mindfulness, and concentration:

Right Effort

This is the will to find peace, prevent evil and unhealthy mental states from arising, as well as the will to eliminate such evil and unhealthy states of the mind that are already risen.

Right mindfulness

This means being consciously aware, attentive, and mindful of your bodily activities, your mind, feelings, or sensations, and finally be aware of thoughts, ideas, things, and conceptions. One way to develop attentiveness of the mind is to practice concentration breathing. When it comes to sensations and feelings, one should be aware of all feelings regardless of them being pleasant or unpleasant and how they appear and disappear. Be aware of all your mind's movements, how they come up and go. When it comes to thoughts and ideas, notice their nature, how they come and go, how they get developed, how they get suppressed and destroyed, and so forth.

Right Concentration

The last factor in mental discipline is developed through the right effort, mindfulness, and concentration is the right concentration. The goal is to have a that mind is disciplined and trained to remain with only equanimity and awareness, even if sensation arise.

Wisdom

In the eightfold path, wisdom is found in the last two factors: right thought and understanding.

Right Thought

True wisdom is found in the noble qualities of selfless detachment, non-violence, and love, while lack of wisdom is associated with thoughts of ill-will, selfishness, and violence in every aspect of life that pollute your mind and make you unhappy.

Right Understanding

Understanding of things the way they really are. This is the pinnacle of wisdom which sees the absolute reality. This understanding is made of knowledge and is only possible when the mind is free of impurities, developed fully, and through meditation.

As you see, the eightfold path, it is a way of life that can be followed and practiced by any person regardless of their religious affiliations. It is a guide to self-discipline of the body, mind and word, self-purification and development, and is not based on any beliefs, prayers, or ceremonies. This is a path that will help you to stop your *Monkey Mind* and your thoughts from jumping uncontrolled and will lead you to embrace happiness, spiritual, moral, and intellectual peace because you won't be having thoughts, saying words and undertaking actions that will result in suffering and unhappiness for yourself and others.

Poisons and medicines of the mind

According to the Buddhist teachings, there are three poisons of the mind:

hatred, greed, and delusion. The metaphors used to describe them are the three fires or three unwholesome roots indicating how dangerous thoughts and emotions can get if not understood and changed.

Greed is the selfishness that lies in the nature of human beings, all the unnecessary desires, the attachments and the cravings for happiness outside of ourselves.

Hatred is related your anger, your repulsion towards unpleasant people or things and circumstances.

Delusion has to do with your dullness and misperception of the real world, basically your wrong reality views.

These three poisons are the result of ignorance about your true nature. These poisonous states of the mind make you develop non-virtuous thoughts, words and actions which translate into suffering and unhappiness.

Unfortunately, these three poisons are deeply rooted in the personality of most people. Your behavior is influenced and tarnished by the three poisons buried in your mind but is also affected by how they influence the others around you. The poisons manifest as lust, anger, cravings, misunderstandings and resentment, and if not checked, they will affect your life in a bad way. Buddha explains how these poisons act like bonds, hindrances, knots or fetters, causing unwholesome karma and all of the human suffering. It is very empowering to understand the three poisons because you will clearly see and feel the causes of confusion, suffering, and unhappiness in your life. With a clear understanding of this, you can now make a decision to get rid of them. According to the teachings of the four noble truths, when you understand the causes of your suffering and dissatisfaction, you can take the action to eliminate them and liberate yourself. Let's study them:

Greed

Greed is that burning desire or craving towards objects o and the need to find a lasting satisfaction in them. This poison creates inside you an inner hunger that makes you always push toward unreachable goals. You wrongfully think that once you attain that goal, you will find happiness and satisfaction that lasts. You may think that if you lose weight you will feel happier, but you forget that to do so you need to use your mind to lose the weight in the right way to succeed and when you fail you feel worst. However, after attaining it, you may not feel that happy because your mind will want something else and you may not find lasting satisfaction. Greed will rise up again to look for the next thing to bring you satisfaction and stress you out until you get it. You will never find contentment because greed will affect every aspect of your life unless you understand your cravings and start controlling your greed. Greed will also flare up as a lack of compassion and generosity for others. It will push you to constantly desire more, better, bigger by wanting to satisfy your insatiable inner hunger and craving.

Hatred

Hatred can manifest itself with different symptoms like anger, revenge, dislike, ill-will, hostility or aversion, wishing harm and suffering for others. Aversion will lead you to resist, avoid, or deny unpleasing feelings, people, or circumstances you are uncomfortable with. We all desire everything to be perfect all the time but it is impossible because we live in impermanent world and there are many things out of our control, like sickness, death, the weather or other people. Hatred and anger will throw you into a cycle of always seeing enemies around you and this bad energy is even able to call them in. When you perceive a likelihood of an enemy around you, your mind is fully occupied with strategies of revenge or protection and cannot remain calm and focus. With hatred, you will find yourself denying and pushing your inner feelings of hurt, loneliness, or fear and treat the feelings as internal enemies. This poison creates conflicts and enemies around you as well as within yourself too.

Delusion

This is your wrong perception or view of reality. Delusion is your misunderstanding and misperception of the workings of the reality you live in. This is perceptional distortion, an inability to understand things as they are. Delusion influences you not to have harmony within yourself and others or with life as a whole. You fight to keep things and relations in a certain way that makes you happy but you forget how live really is. Delusion arises from ignorance to the true nature of reality and your own true nature. This means that you constantly search outside yourself for happiness and solutions to your problems. Delusion makes you unable to perceive which actions are the root of your happiness and which non-virtuous and unhealthy deeds cause you suffering. Delusion binds you to a place where you don't seem to find a way out.

Medicines of the mind

After talking about the poison and the problems of the mind, we can now start studying the solutions. By now, you may have realized that your life has been motivated and influenced by the three poisons and the first step to get rid of them is to identify and analyze them. In order to purify and transform your mind, you must be patient. It requires care, persistence, patience, and deep compassion for others as well as yourself. According to Buddha, the poisons of the mind that cause so much suffering can be transformed and purified. It is indeed possible for you to break negative karma and suffering and live a fulfilled happy life. Buddha further says that our true nature is that of enlightenment, liberation and it can naturally shine through if you have a purified mind and heart. Therefore, the purpose of your spiritual practice is to free yourself from the things that obscure the nature of radiance, clarity, and the joy of your enlightenment. So how do you face the three poisons and change them in a way of true freedom?

The work of purification must start from the origin of the poisons, the mind.

You have to learn to calm your mind and deeply explore within yourself. This simply means that you must first recognize the three poisons within yourself, when they appear and disappear and how they do affect your mind your thoughts, your feelings and definitively, your life. When you become consciously aware of them, you are then able to discern how they negatively influence your reactions, thoughts, speech, actions, and feelings, so you are ready for the second step which is understanding your ability to transform them. To do this, you will have to train your mind to meditate, concentrate on your breathing allowing your thoughts to come and go without reactions towards them. Do not worry, you will find how to do it in the following chapters of this book. Practicing the exercises that I will show you later, you will be able to notice when the thoughts and emotions occur and stop them before they overwhelm you and cause harm to you or those around you.

Antidotes

Apart from meditation, there are also antidotes or alternatives. For every poison, the Buddha has given us a solution or a method to get rid of it and replace these mental attitudes with virtuous thoughts and happier results. The purpose of these antidotes is to get rid of the poisons by cultivating alternative mindsets.

To overcome greed, learn to cultivate selflessness, detachment, contentment, and generosity. If you experience greed, try and think of the disadvantages of your object of desire. Also, try and give out those things you want to hold on to but have become useless for you, declutter. Charity and selfless service to others expecting nothing back will also help you overcome greed. Please note that there is nothing wrong with sharing and enjoying things, but the problem arises when you wrongly attach to things o persons and start believing that the source of your happiness is outside yourself.

In order to overcome hatred, learn to cultivate loving kindness, patience, forgiveness, and compassion. Learn to meet your own unpleasant experiences or circumstances with patience, understanding that they are teaching you a lesson, do it compassion, and kindness to yourself and others. When you experience feelings of insecurity, hurt, doubt, and so forth, analyze your thoughts and practice openness with someone who knows you and you trust to have another point of view, and always be kind to yourself. Thank yourself for starting this transformation and forgive yourself for everything that happened in your past due to your uncontrolled mind. Your will notice that this practice will open your heart and let go of hatred.

To overcome delusion, you will need to cultivate wisdom, to get a right understanding of reality, and insight in your true nature. Embrace reality as it is and avoid distorting it with your desires, expectations and fears. Seek to understand the nature of impermanence, of this ever-changing world realizing that you can't control everything, that the creation is interrelated and that lasting happiness comes from within not from without. Understand which are the positive and healthy actions that bring you happiness as well as the negative ones that cause you suffering and avoid them. Aim to cultivate insight, right understanding, and wisdom and be free from the delusions of your mind.

If you carefully apply the teachings of Buddha, you will slowly eradicate your uncontrolled mind, thoughts and all the behaviors that are not good for you and you will be finally free from stress, suffering and unhappiness. When you finally start liberating your mind from the three poisons of the mind, peace, bliss, and wisdom will shine through. Remember that it is our nature to be happy and that we all have the potential of complete liberation.

"All the suffering in the world comes from selfishness,
all the happiness in the world comes from
compassion".

Shantideva

THE EIGHT VERSES OF THOUGHT TRANSFORMATION

Shantideva was an 8th-century Indian Buddhist Monk and scholar that apparently was one of those people who didn't appear to study much or practice meditation sessions. His fellow monks said that his three "realizations" were eating, sleeping, and shitting, but after being goaded into addressing the entire university body, Shantideva surprised everyone with speech that became famous and was recollected in a book called *"The way of the Bodhisattva"*, which I really recommend you to read as it treats the awakening of the mind. But for now let us pay attention to his *"Eight verses of thought transformation"* that are based in love and compassion. Remember that working consistently with logical reasoning and analysis, will enable you to change your mind or attitude into a truer and better you.

I - Focused to acquire the greatest benefit for all living beings who are more important than a wish giving jewel, I shall hold them close at all times.

We all want to be happy and free and this need equalizes all living beings. This verse is based on two attitudes; that of selfishly cherishing your and cherishing others. The selfish attitude makes you uptight, thinking that you are more important than others, give you a narrow view with the selfish desire to find happiness for only yourself. Self-cherishing attitude, however, does not bring you happiness, but stress as you always have to work on cherishing yourself. When you start putting your attention on others above yourself and regard them as important as you are, you will be surprised at how happy you become. If you try to help others, you are likely to experience joy and receive good feelings back of love from those you help. Your mind will stop going around your problems and desires all the time and it will give you a rest. The bottom line of this verse simply states that a selfish attitude will just bring you separation and loneliness.

II - When in the company of others, I shall always consider myself the lowest of all, and from the depths of my heart hold others dear and supreme.

Regardless of who you find yourself with, thoughts of superiority may arise in you generating pride within. This attitude, as I already explained to you is delusional, try instead to cultivate yourself in being humble. Note that helping others does not make you better than them, so be humble because you do not know of their burdens. Be grateful that you have the opportunity to train your mind by helping them and get the rewards of it.

III - I will be vigilant, and the moment a delusion appears in my mind, endangering myself and others, I shall confront and avert it without delay.

If the negative thoughts should arise investigate the causes in your mind. Remember that identifying and understanding them lowers theirs powers to stop the disturbing negative mind, try to recite a mantra, like the ones I showed you before, and mediate on impermanence, anger, attachment or death.

IV - Whenever I see beings that are wicked in nature and overwhelmed by violent negative actions and suffering, I shall hold such rare ones dear, as if I had found a precious treasure.

When you should come across nasty, cruel, rough, or unpleasant people, our usual reaction is to avoid him. In such situations our loving concern for others is liable to decrease. Instead of allowing our love for others to weaken by thinking what an evil person he is, we should see him as a special object of love and compassion and cherish that person as though we had come across a precious treasure, difficult to find.

V - When, out of envy, others mistreat me with abuse, insults or the like, I shall accept defeat and offer the victory to others.

When you encounter a person that criticizes and abuses you claiming you are incompetent you are likely to get very angry and contradict what the person has said. We should not react in this way; instead, with humility and tolerance, we should accept what has been said. But if somebody is doing something harmful and dangerous to another living being it is wrong not to take the necessary measures to stop it. The motivation should not be a selfish concern but extensive feelings of kindness and compassion towards others.

VI - When someone I have helped and in whom I have high expectations of hurts me, I shall regard them as my teacher.

This verse talks about patience. It is normal for you to expect gratitude from those that you have helped but in case they show no gratitude in their interactions with you, you should not get angry. Practice patience and compassion in such a situation and see them as teachers trying your patience and so treat them respectively.

VII - In short, both directly and indirectly, I offer every happiness and benefit to all my mothers. I shall secretly take upon myself all their harmful actions and suffering.

This refers to the practice of giving others happiness while we carry their burdens. This is motivated by love and compassion. Just as we desire happiness, all the other beings desire the same too. When we see others suffering and we notice that they are overwhelmed by suffering but do not know how to get rid of it, we should secretly generate the intention of taking on all their suffering.

VII - Undefiled by the stains of the superstitions of the eight worldly concerns, may I, by perceiving all phenomena as illusory, be released from the bondage of attachment.

In these verse Shantideva talks about wisdom and not allowing all the practices to be negatively influenced by superstitions. We have to start recognizing all existence as illusory and, in this way, one can be liberated from the bondage of this type of clinging Mediate in emptiness and you will understand that objects are devoid of true existence.

To this point, I hope you have acknowledged the importance of understanding your own human mind and the way and reason your thoughts and feelings arise, as well as the need for you to control your mind and your thoughts. Only if you start doing it, will you be able to change your life for better and settle for your goals. Remember that you are not your mind, and that by playing with it, you can get control of your thoughts. We will see how in following chapters.

CHAPTER THREE

INVESTIGATE YOUR PAST

Y our past has a direct influence on your present life. In this chapter, I will show you how your past influences your feelings, thoughts and actions and how to handle your past presently.

YOUR PAST AFFECTS YOUR PRESENT

When you embark on a journey to find the real you in order to live a happier and fulfilling life, you will need to investigate, understand and forgive anything that happened in the past. Even if you do not realize you are carrying the burden of your past experiences, because even if you do not recall any traumatic experience they have made you as you are now. Your personality and behavior today is the result of what you have lived. Everything that happened in your childhood, in your teenager years or even last month have built the self you are now. Your family, teachers, friends, work, what you read or watch in TV all of that is part of the clutter in your past. That does not mean that is all bad, what I want you to understand is that what you have lived has made you as you are now and revisiting it will help you to understand yourself and cure any pain that you may be carrying. All events regardless of how big or small they were, are likely to affect your current life and your future.

Clutter in your past can act as the obstacles in today's life, hindering you from moving forward. Your actual feelings and thoughts are likely to have been influenced by your past experiences as well as the way you act or interact with people today may be as a result of events in your childhood or young adulthood life.

It is important that you understand the relation between your present and your past and how your past will influence your future.

When a child is born starts collecting information from their environment, their family ways and believes setting up the basis of that child's life. Psychologists say that children are able to absorb information so fast, that by the age of 6 years, they have formed their core beliefs. The beliefs that you formed in your earlier life are likely to influence you negatively or positively, but is important to acknowledge them so you accept them again. Please note that it is possible to change any negative experiences and beliefs and transform your life. You will have to face all the ghosts and skeletons that you keep inside and try to hide, but know that it is the only way you can free yourself from them. If you don't do it, they will keep tormenting you for the rest of your life. It will take courage a lot of patience and discipline, but I guaranty you that it is the best think you can do for yourself and your future.

Change your beliefs to change your personality

You may ask yourself how is it possible to change your beliefs. First, begin by acknowledging the beliefs that have moulded your personality over the years. After establishing them, it is time to dig into your past and identify what led you to form those beliefs. This is not easy to do because as the beliefs were getting formed, you may not have been aware hence you feel powerless over them. However, once you are able to get to the root of why you formed certain beliefs, it gets easier to deal with them. Identifying and understanding how they were formed is what gives you the power to break free from their hold. To understand it better, consider the following scene: Suppose your boss complains that your performance was below average and you did not deliver as expected and that he expects better performance in the new month. Will you want to know what went wrong and how it happened so as to fix it? The same way in your behavior, if you don't understand what caused you to behave in a certain way, then it will be impossible to change it. This is the main reason why in order to change and start living a better life free of useless clutter, you must identify the past clutter of the mind, how it was formed and where it came from, so you can deal with it and conclusively declutter and free yourself. These few illustrations serve to show you how your past can shape your present:

If a you grew up in a household that was violent, where you may grow up believing that this is the normal behavior. It is likely that you become abusive or submissive in your relations because it is the way your learned growing up. In case that you suffered abuse (physically or mentally) as a child or a teen, even if you don't remember it now, it can have affected your self-esteem. Later life, you may develop a shy and frighten personality that may stop you from following any goals, or not even have them. On the other side, if you received a lot of attention growing up, you have the danger to develop the need to be always recognized. In adulthood, this need for attention can translate in selfishness and laziness.

The above examples are just to explain how experiences in the past can cause a person to develop unknowingly certain behaviors and beliefs, and affect the character.

If you truly desire to change your life for better, you need to purpose to declutter your mind from the past and the negative beliefs. This also applies to phobias and fears because if you were attacked by an animal or someone told you that rats or cockroach are dirty and bring illness, or you were left in the dark and got really scared, you may very well have had a trauma from this experience and still carry it in your subconscious, even though you do not remember when and how it was generated. This is why is so important to know your past so you can create your present.

The shadow according to Carl Jung

Carl Jung was a Swiss psychologist who developed the concept of the *'shadow'* inside us. He described it as those parts of one's personality that a person has suppressed or rejected unconscionably. Every individual has aspects of themselves that are not liked and so they are pushed down to unconscious psyches building a collection of the suppressed areas of one's identity. You may think you love yourself the way you are or there is nothing wrong with you, but the truth is you also may not be aware of the parts of your personality that you have rejected and how they influence your present life.

Your mind will try to ignore them instead of confronting them but they still live inside you and the deeper rooted the more their influence in you. Some of the shadows include shameful experiences, immoral urges, aggressive impulses, unacceptable sexual fantasies, irrational wishes and fears. These aspects even though buried deep into your subconscious and unacknowledged by you are the ones shaping your personality and character. You may see all the faults you have in others but not in yourself. You have to see the others as the mirror of yourself. What you do not like in others is what you hate in yourself. Here are some examples:

Judgment of others especially on impulse

You see someone walking down the street and you immediately comment how ridiculous their outfit looks. You perceive yourself as better and smarter than the person and because you would not like to be singled out yourself, you use this as a way to reassure yourself.

Seeing your insecurities as flaws in others

This can best be seen through the behaviors of internet trolls. They hide behind the keyboard and comment on people's posts with negative words maybe because the comment has touched a nerve in them.

Quick temper with subordinates
Some people find it easier to exercise their power over those that can't fight back. This habit is a way of replacing one's feelings of defeat when faced by a greater force.

According to Jung, it is very difficult to see the shadow or the dark side in yourself, because is easier to see the dark or the shadow in others. These suppressed aspects influence and control your behavior and are the reason why you react the way you do. Some of these aspects are very poisonous to your mind and are a heavy burden to you because you have not acknowledged them. You must then seek to free yourself from these dark or shadow aspects in order to life a better life. Jung suggests to do the *'shadow work'* to bring the dark or the shadow inside you into light. It is important to note that whatever you suppress does not disappear but stays in your unconscious and most of your behavior is controlled by the unconscious. Shadow work is the process of bringing the unconscious to the conscious in order for you to acknowledge, understand and accept it, so you are finally able to take control of your own life.

Meditation is the way to begin this process of shadow work as it helps you to look within yourself and identify the shadow aspects. The next step would be to identify the triggers of the reactions that are responsible for you to behave in a way that is not favorable to you. It is the only way you learn to deal with aspects of your past that influence your present life and help you to live better.

If you want to overcome some challenges you are facing now, you need to investigate your past, understand what shapes your behavior today so you will identify what needs to be changed and how to change it. If you want to declutter yourself and live better, then the best place to begin is your past. Dig through your unconscious mind and discover some suppressed aspects of yourself, bring them out, and deal with them to overcome them and find freedom.

Now I am going to explain you some techniques that can help you do the shadow work. You can try to do it by yourself but in my experience sometimes is good to look for the help of a professional. My recommendation is that you investigate in the following technics and then chose one that you find more suitable for you.

ENNEAGRAMS

The Enneagram is a personality grouping system. Every person is considered to belong to one type or group, but it is possible to have characteristics of another types. The Enneagram is described as a model of the human psyche which is divided in nine interconnected personality types or *'enneatypes'*. Its origins can be found in George Gurdjieff teachings and have been developed by Oscar Ichazo and Claudio Naranjo.

There are nine enneagram types represented by numbers 1 to 9, and as I said before each of them with different trait and characteristics. Everyone has a dominant trait that was established early in your life. The nine personality types are represented by the points of a geometric figure called enneagram (*see below*) and indicate connections between the types. The enneagram figure is usually composed of three parts: a circle that represents unity, an inner triangle and an irregular hexagon. It is illustrated by a circle that has arrows pointing in different directions. In addition to the main type, there is a dominant wing which is usually on either side of the main type.

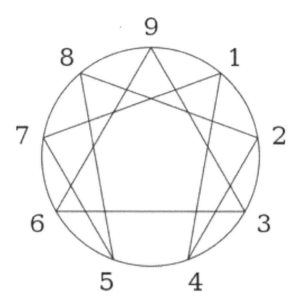

To find out which is your enneagram type you can find enneagram tests in Internet. Here I will explain you some of the main qualities and negative traits of each one. In case you want to follow this technique I recommend you to look for a professional as the enneagram has influences from other types and they can be very important. Enneagram can help you to understand your personality and your past, because it is a way into your subconscious mind.

The nine enneagrams are:

Type 1 - The Reformer

The Rational, Idealistic Type: Principled, Purposeful, Self-Controlled, and Perfectionistic

This personality trait is based on the desire to make everything better because nothing seems to be good enough. This personality type would belong to a perfectionist with a high sense of responsibility and obsessed with improvements. They desire to make order everywhere they go. These people normally hold on resentment even anger because they have some kind of imbalance inside themselves. The can become hypocrites and fall in hypercriticism of selves and others.

Type 2 - The Helper

The Caring, Interpersonal Type: Demonstrative, Generous, People-Pleasing, and Possessive

The persons under the type 2 of the enneagram are selfless, generous and giving, socially involved and most of them extroverts. They are eager to please and go out of their way to help anyone in need because they like flattery. As they measure their own worth by the ability for others to need their help they try to be needed at all times. Their desire to be loved can make them forget their own needs and suffer manipulation from others.

Type 3 - The Achiever

The Success-Oriented, Pragmatic Type: Adaptive, Excelling, Driven, and Image-Conscious

For them to find validation, their focus is in the image of success because their main fear is to feel worthless. They desire to be admired and can become vain and conceited. These people follow the laws and are usually hard workers, competitive, and focused on the attainment of their goals because they always stress themselves to be better.

Type 4 - The Individualist

The Sensitive, Withdrawn Type: Expressive, Dramatic, Self-Absorbed, and Temperamental

They build their personality around the belief that they are different and unique. They are very individualistic and perceive their difference from others as both a gift and a curse. These people hold themselves as unique and different from the rest to the point that they can feel unable to enjoy and find happiness in what others enjoy.

Type 5 - The Investigator

The Intense, Cerebral Type: Perceptive, Innovative, Secretive, and Isolated

This type doubts the own inner strength to face life and so feels often withdrawn. They find safety and security in their mind as they think of strategies of how they can face the world that is why they try to replace direct experience with concepts. They are intelligent, well educated, very thoughtful, and often become experts in areas that interest them.

Type 6 - The Loyalist

The Committed, Security-Oriented Type: Engaging, Responsible, Anxious, and Suspicious

They are usually very insecure and fear to be left without support and guidance. They don't trust easily, they are fearful and anxious. They are usually doubtful of others until one proves themselves trustworthy and once they trust, they are totally loyal to the person. They should find faith in themselves to avoid depending in external reassurance.

Type 7 - The Enthusiast

The Busy, Fun-Loving Type: Spontaneous, Versatile, Distractible, and Scattered

They seek fun and adventure in their lives. They are always looking into the future believing better things are just about to happen. They are very energetic, great thinkers, and planners. These people are extroverts, creative, talented in different areas, and open-minded. They fear deprivation and are always trying to feel satisfied and content, that is why they may tend to gluttony.

Type 8 - The Challenger

The Powerful, Dominating Type: Self-Confident, Decisive, Willful, and Confrontational

They are often controlling or masters of their own fate and fear being harmed, controlled and dominated by others. They are energetic, strong-willed, tough-minded, decisive, and practical. They are often overpowering or domineering and that can affect the relations with others who do not want to be dominated. They seek truth and can be vengeful.

Type 9 - The Peacemaker

The Easy-going, Self-Effacing Type: Receptive, Reassuring, Agreeable, and Complacent

They avoid conflict as much as they can. They focus on peace and harmony in every aspect of their lives that is why they keep to themselves, thus they are often introverted. They fear loss, fragmentation and separation. Some of them may be active in their social lives but only to some degree as they protect themselves from the possibility of conflict.

How enneagrams help you cure your past

The Enneagram of personality is important for anyone seeking to take their personal growth to a new level. Enneagram helps you to bring awareness of your unconscious need and understand the strategies you use to meet those needs. It opens the door to acknowledge your own personality and the characteristics more intimately. Once you know your enneagram type, you can see the extremes of your personality and what you can do to deal with your negative trails and improve the positive ones.

Enneagram will help you to increase your capacity for self-reflection. It will give you a vision of the manifestation of the best you as well as your average and worst. For instance, if we look at type seven, at its healthiest, it appreciates experiences deeply, hence becoming extremely grateful and appreciative. They are amazed by small wonders in life, are joyful and excited about life. At average manifestation, the personality trait exhibits restlessness desiring to have more choices or options. They may become adventurous but less focused, always looking for new experiences and things and keeping up with trends. At the extreme of unhealthy, they may become desperate to calm their anxieties and can easily fall into addictions that dominate them without knowing how to stop. They can also be very offensive and abusive.

Every enneagram has a passion. This passion is what drives the personality to satisfy its needs. Enneagrams can help you recognize when your passions have taken over, hence helping you establish how to satisfy your needs in a healthy way. Every passion can be turned into a virtue once you understand it. For sevens, the unhealthy passion is gluttony with the virtue being sobriety. When you are aware of your passion of gluttony, then you can work on transforming it to sobriety. The passions and virtues of enneagrams are:

- Type 1 - passion: anger, resentment / virtue: serenity
- Type 2 - passion: pride / virtue: humility
- Type 3 - passion: vanity or deceit / virtue: integrity
- Type 4 - passion: envy / virtue: equanimity or acceptance
- Type 5 - passion: avarice or greed / virtue: generosity
- Type 6 - passion: fear or anxiety / virtue: courage
- Type 7 - passion: gluttony / virtue: sobriety
- Type 8 - passion: intensity / virtue: innocence or surrender
- Type 9 - passion: indifference / virtue: engagement or action

As you can see, your behavior and character can highly be influenced by your type of enneagram. Once you know your personality type or enneagram, you will be able to understand what pushes you to behave the way you do and what are your basic goals in life. Enneagrams enable you to deeply look within yourself and establish your behavior patterns, what triggers certain behaviors, and how to change your behavior for better. For instance, if you are a five, you may find that you have been driven by greed which is your personality passion in order to heal you should choose to purposely cultivate your virtue which is generosity. When you kill the negative traits by making your virtues stronger, you find healing and you become a better truer version of you.

AYAHUASCA

Ayahuasca is a sacred plant brew medicine used by cultures in the Amazon for thousands of years. Ayahuasca is a sacred and powerful medicine used for spiritual awakening, healing and even divination. It is not a drug and is not addictive but it should be treated with great respect. The indigenous people around the Amazon often give this powerful medicine to their children from a very young age. Ayahuasca has huge potential for healing the psychological levels as well as the physical. A master plant, she is also referred to as Mother Ayahuasca because of her teaching and healing effects. Ayahuasca is a vine called *Banisteriopsis Caapi* which grows in the Amazon Rainforest and has mainly no psychotropic effect. To produce the powerful medicine, the vine has to be boiled together with leaves of the Chacruna shrub or *Psychotria virdis*. For this purpose, the vine is pulled apart into thin strips and then cooked together with the Chacruna leaves in a pot with water for several days until it becomes a thick liquid. The resulting potion is then the medicine and has a strong bitter taste.

Working with ayahuasca has been described as deep, profound, and very transformative. It is an experience that facilitates deep healing in every aspect of a human being; physical, emotional, spiritual and mental. It allows access to your higher state of consciousness and an experience of spiritual awakening. You should never take Ayahuasca without the guiding of a professional with experience in the field. Nowadays some phycologists use it in their therapies but you can also try it with a trustful healer with renown. Before you try it, please talk to someone who has already experienced an ayahuasca retreat for advice. You do not need to travel to Brazil or to the depths of the Amazonas, it is better if your first experience is near home with people who have the necessary knowledge and work with the right medicine, and that, at any time, before, during and after your retreat, will be there to help you in your process and the integration of new knowledge.

Benefits of Ayahuasca

The benefits of Ayahuasca vary from person to person. Remember that the use of Ayahuasca should be therapeutic and done by a professional in order to benefit your physical and mental health. Some psychologist and psychiatrists use Ayahuasca because of the benefits experienced by persons that have taken this substance that include emotional cleanse, reduction of anxiety, or addiction and depression recovery. Ayahuasca can to expand your awareness, help you to get deep into your mind and find answers and motives many things that you are not consciously aware of.

Ayahuasca Ceremony

Before we continue, I strongly advise anyone who does not have experience with Ayahuasca not to take this medicine without being well informed by a practitioner with experience. There are many associations that offer these ceremonies but please, if you decide to try it, do it under the guidance of recognized professional. In addition to the effects, such as vomiting and diarrhea, strong visions can also occur, which can lead to anxiety if one does not know how to deal with it. Therefore, it is extremely important that the ceremony be carried out with a skilled psychologist or shaman, who can intervene and help in such a case.

The ayahuasca ceremony begins with the shaman, the person guiding the ceremony, offering a prayer for the protection of the ceremony by inviting the right energy spirit for the work, praying for each persons' purpose in the ceremony as well. Every person is expected to focus on their intention and purpose during the prayer.

After the prayers, everyone is given the medicine The shaman sings medicine songs, so-called Icaro chants ushering in the energy of the medicine. Peaceful tranquility sets in as the ceremony continue. The speed at which the medicine comes varies. For some, it can be 15 minutes and for others, even an hour. Some people may vomit and others may purge through other ways like yawning, tears, breathing, and a release of obsessive thoughts thus removing the old energy from within yourself. The Ayahuasca ceremony is not conducted in total darkness, a fire is made that provides light and when the ceremony has progressed and all are comfortable, the fire may be reduced in order to create ambience. This is the moment where everyone is quietly focusing on their journey. Then a second cup of ayahuasca is given to those that still need it. Please note that different people require different amounts of medicine. Whether you vomit, have diarrhea or get visions depends on the individual person and therefore it is impossible to tell someone what will happen to them during a ceremony. In the right setting and under the right guidance, however, the medicine can be taken without hesitation and without any risk. After five hours everyone's journey is coming to a close and the shaman starts the closing prayer thanksgiving for water, life, and food. Once the ceremony is ended the participants have breakfast and get some rest. Hours after everyone is gathered together to share the experience and have the counsel of the shaman.

CONSTELLATIONS

You we born into family, culture and society and yet you are an individual. You have to live combing both the personal and social aspects of yourself simultaneously. Your entry into the world is your first experience of others and provides an initial impression of who you are through their eyes. Through this you have formed a deep psychological imprint of who you are. It forms your idea of self-worth. The problem is if these early bonds are not formed well because you will carry them into adulthood. You take this evaluation of ourselves into the world. Self-esteem is the core foundation for worthiness and our choices in relationships, career, success and wellbeing. Feelings such as sadness are easily passed through generations via relational bonds. If how you feel about yourself is due to our early bonding or family patterns, don't you think that the family system is a fundamental issue to explore?

Family Constellations are also known as Systemic Constellations and are a therapeutic method used to heal the past. The scope of the family constellations is to reveal an unrecognized dynamic that has been occurring for generations in a given family and to cure the negative and harmful effects of that dynamic by encouraging the person, through representatives, to encounter and accept the factual reality of the past. Family constellations are an effective method to transform whatever is unconsciously stagnating you and blocking you from living your life according to your greatest potential. Their purpose is to enable you to break existing poisonous patterns that have been happening in your family for many generations.

The idea is that present-day problems and difficulties may be influenced by traumas suffered in previous generations of the family, even if those affected now are unaware of the original event. They are not caused by direct personal experience but have occurred in the past producing unresolved trauma has afflicted different generations of a family. This are usually traumatic events such as murder, suicide, death of a mother in childbirth, early death of a parent or sibling, war, natural disaster, abortion, emigration, or abuse.

Familial bonds certainly can have an influence on your mental well-being, whether it's your biological family or the family you create on your own. You depend on them for advice, emotional support or even as a resource for your troubles. Plus, you plan your life and future with them.

Benefits of Family Constellations

This technique can help you to understand and transform your past. It exposes cross-generational dynamics that are hidden but still unconsciously affect your life. Empowers and enhances your relationships and your ability to respond to challenges. You can become aware of your self-sabotage and blockages and transform them.

Clinical experience also shows that family constellation therapy can be used to help a number of conditions like recurring negative emotions such as fear, depression, anxiety; self-sabotage; problems in relationships; addictions;

unknown or unexplained health symptoms; problems achieving life goals.

The Method of Family Constellations

The Family Constellations are celebrated as a workshop with a group of different people that are led by a facilitator. In turn, members of the group will be given the opportunity explore personal issues. The facilitator will establish which members of the group are to participate in the Constellation. The person presenting the issue is called the seeker and he/she will ask other members of the group to join the Constellation as representatives. He or she will arrange these representatives according to what feels right in the moment. The seeker then sits down and observes the behavior of the selected persons that intuitively will mirror those of the real family members they represent. They will be asked how they feel being placed in relation to the others that will show the dynamic that influences the issue that it is treated. The facilitator will ask questions and makes changes adding more members to the constellation until the facilitator feels that the healing resolution has taken hold among the representatives. Then, the seeker is invited to take the place of his/her representative in the Constellation and perceive the new reconfigured system. The Constellation concludes once everyone feels comfortable in their place meaning that the healing has taken place.

TEMAZCAL

Temazcal are sweat lodges used in Mexico since ancient times. A temazcal is a structure constructed from volcanic rock and is usually built in a dome shape. It is like a modern steam room. The name translates as "house of heat" and the ceremonies held inside are considered to be healing and purification ceremonies that cleanse the mind, body, and spirit.

The heat is produced from heated volcanic rocks that are put in a pit at the center or by the wall of a temazcal. This sweat room or lodge was used in ancient Mesoamerica during curative ceremonies to purify the body activities like a battle but also as a place for women to give birth, heal the sick, or improve one's health.

Ceremony

Temazcal ceremonies or rituals are extremely hot. The ceremony is typically carried out for small groups by a shaman who's usually a member of one of the Mayan communities. The process lasts around two hours and entails entering the temazcal with little or no clothing on and sweating it out to the sound of chanting and the fragrance of herbs. Anyone with diabetes or heart disease should restrain from the ceremony, while those susceptible to claustrophobia might think twice before they participate as once you get in you won't be able to leave unless you have the permission of the shaman. Note that the door will be closed with a thick blanket and the only light you will see is the sparks of the rocks when the water is poured on them. During the session the shaman will pour through water, rosemary, basil, peppermint and other scents over the pile of hot rocks in a pit in the middle of the floor to create vapor. Note that the temazcal represents the sacred "womb" of Mother Earth.

To begin, the Shaman will gather the participants to give respect to the 6 directions, north, south, east, west, sky, and earth. The first step before entering the temazcal is a cleansing with a traditional tree resin, Copal. The Shaman will "smudge" you or blow this smoke over your body to chase away any negative energies before you enter in order to allow the healing enter more easily. The doorway is small so you will need to kneel to enter the dark chamber. As you kneel, you will touch your forehead to the ground and say: *"To all my relations"*, a reverence to your guides and ancestors. From there, you will enter, always clockwise, all the way around the fire pit to sit closely, cross legged, knee to knee with your neighbor. The shaman will start drumming and will continue until there is total concentration. Then he/she will ask the participants for their intention to attend the ceremony and direct everyone to let emotions, fears, heaviness, and bad energy to go out with the smoke, steam, vapor, and music as the blanket over the doorway is removed.

There will be four sessions or "*Puertas*" (doors), one for each direction. This means every 15-30 minutes the door will open and new hot stone or "grandmother" will be passed in for the next session. As the last door is ending, you will give thanks to the experience and everyone involved and then exit counter clockwise out of the symbolic "womb" created by the temazcal.

Benefits of Temazcal

One of the physical benefits of a temazcal ceremony is detoxifying the body. Due to the high temperatures the body releases toxins through sweating cleansing the body from impurities. The steamy ritual with herbs, especially mint relieves symptoms of cold and clears any blockages. Patients with chronic fatigue syndrome have found that exposure to high temperatures significantly reduces fatigue, insomnia, and pain. It can also relieve arthritis and improves endurance, mental performance and resilience.

HYPNOTHERAPY

Hypnotherapy is a therapy in which the mind is used to help with a variety of problems, such as breaking bad habits or coping with fear, anxiety or stress. The job of the hypnotherapist is to induce hypnotic state in a patient in order to increase motivation or alter harmful behavioral patterns. The professional will consults with client to determine nature of problem and how it affects him/her and the client to enter hypnotic state by explaining how hypnosis works and what client will experience.

Hypnosis or hypnotherapy uses guided relaxation, intense concentration, and focused attention to achieve a heightened state of awareness. The person's attention is so focused while in this state that anything going on around the person is temporarily blocked out or ignored. It is usually considered an aid to physiotherapy because the hypnotic state allows people to explore painful thoughts, feelings, and memories they might have hidden from their conscious minds. In addition, hypnosis enables people to perceive some things differently, such as blocking an awareness of pain. The hypnotic state makes the person better able to respond to suggestions, so guided by a professional it can help to change certain behaviors, such as additions, the perceptions of fear and sensations of anxiety, and is particularly useful in treating pain. It also helps to explore a possible psychological root cause of a disorder or symptom caused by a traumatic past event that a person has hidden in his or her unconscious memory. Once the trauma is revealed, it can be addressed and cured.

You can also learn how to do it yourself learning self-hypnosis conditioning.

Benefits of Hypnotherapy

Hypnotherapy can help you transform your eating behaviors and drop pounds or stop smoking – It helps smokers stop the habit of smoking. Unwanted patterns of behavior that may lead to depression can be changed by the combination of hypnosis and cognitive-behavioral change, hypnotherapy. It has been used on people with severe chronic pain and they find relief. Because of relaxation, hypnosis was found to improve sleep patterns in people suffering from insomnia.

VIPASSANA

Vipassana is the oldest of the Buddhist practices of meditation for the cultivation of awareness and mindfulness and has been used as a universal remedy for universal ills. It means *'to see things as they really are'*. It is a method of self-transformation through self-observation. It focuses on the deep interconnection between mind and body based on self-exploratory journey that helps the practitioner to understand his/her feelings, judgements and sensations, and through this experience, how the own mind works. That is why learning Vipassana will increase your awareness as well as learn self-control and how to find your inner peace.

It is a system that trains your mind through a set of exercises directed to help you become more aware of your own life experiences. Note that this is a gradual process that can take longer than a ten days retreat, in fact, years, but with time, it is possible to break through that wall of delusion. Once this is done, the transformation is complete because the freedom or liberation is permanent.

This technique is taught at ten-day residential course or Vipassana Retreat during which participants learn the basics of the method, and practice sufficiently to experience its beneficial results. The course requires hard and serious work and involve a meditation period of at least 10 hours a day. The noble silence is a vow taken on the first day as you start the retreat. This means no communication with anyone orally or non-verbally. The reason for the silence is to help you focus more and experience the goings on within you. The days start at 4 am to 10 pm, so you will have plenty of time for self-reflection. The sitting position while meditating is uncomfortable at the beginning but as you move along, it will get better and you develop a good sitting posture. During the retreat or the period of the course, you will have to abstain from killing, stealing, sexual activity, speaking falsely, and intoxicants because it serves to calm the mind and allows the self-observation. Men and women are separated for the same reason. You will learn to fix your attention on the flow of your breath paying attention as it enters and leaves the nostrils. Once your mind is calmer and more focused, you will be introduced to the practice of Vipassana itself: observing sensations throughout the body, understanding their nature, and developing equanimity by learning not to react to them. The retreat closes on the tenth day with a meditation on loving kindness or goodwill towards all, in which the purity developed during the course is shared with all beings.

The entire practice is actually a mental training. Just as we use physical exercises to improve our bodily health, Vipassana can be used to develop a healthy mind.

Benefits of a Vipassana retreat

Thanks to the techniques you learn, you begin to be more alert of your personality, the positive and negative sides and more in tune with your emotions. This is the first step to understand, accept and control yourself. The main teaching of Vipassana is equanimity, which is the ability to accept all outcomes be they good or bad. This means that you should enjoy the good times and accept the bad times as lessons, but not get attached to neither, just accept them as a part of life. All temporal things, whether material or mental, only lasts for a limited period of time. Everything is formed of compounded objects in a continuous change of condition, subject to decline and destruction. This is the reason why you should not cling on to people, places or possessions because nothing is permanent. As you observe the noble silence, you are not allowed to read or write or even use cell phones. All your days are spent in deep meditation while keeping distractions away. The lack of distractions allows for deeper meditation and a better detox for the mind. You will have learnt to redirect your mind and stop those disturbing thoughts and redirect your attention to your breath. This will build willpower and perseverance and you will become comfortable in redirecting and guiding your mind towards your goals.

You will come out of the retreat calmer. The ten days of meditation without external distractions helps calm you down. Also, learning to accept things as they are will help you face any situation with a new sense of calmness which will allow you to take better decisions. You have been used to look outside yourself for the causes of your problems but after this retreat you have learned to look within yourself and the manifestations of your own thoughts which will allow you to have a broader view of life.

If you feel attracted to this method, do not hesitate to try it, because, even if it is thought it brings many benefits. Remember that if you should decide to experience a Vipassana retreat, you should attend an approved center where you will be led by professionals.

PSYCHOLOGY

We all have a past that affects us being it traumatic or nor, it needs to be acknowledged and understood. Past experiences are known to influence your present life your character and behavior. Be you cannot live in the past and you cannot carry your painful experiences as a burden with you. They stop you and they put you down, so the best way to get rid of them is to work on your past.

Your current feelings, your personality traits and your current behavior were shaped by the past events you have been through. All the experiences that you have lived, as good or bad as they have been, are dramatically impacting your life right now, even the ones that might seem irrelevant or insignificant, and they will keep affecting your future as long as you don't become aware of the connection between your past and your future. The impact your past has on your present is extremely powerful and unless you learn to understand it and accept it, your whole life might be impacted in a bad way. Some people with past traumatic experiences do not understand the actual reactions and behaviors because they have suppressed those experiences in order to mitigate or reduce the pain. But they still carry this pain as a burden and it can translate in destructive behaviors like overeating, anger issues, drinking, isolation, and many more. Healing is not easy, however, it is possible and doable. Here are a few steps or strategies that will help you in to start this path:

Evaluate your experiences and forgive yourself

Face your past with courage and don't try to deny it. Allow yourself to bring back and be open to thoughts, inner experiences, and feelings from your past. You can do it by yourself but you can also look for the help of a professional. Write down those experiences in a list where you have the good ones in one side and the traumatic ones. Pick an aspect of your experience and meditate on it and notice what it makes you feel. You may notice you experience varied feelings or emotions towards it, written them down too. This will help you increase your awareness of your past history. Whenever you meditate in one of the issues, please say out loud:

> *"Dear memories, replaying in my mind, with gratitude*
> *I let you go, for you and for me. Please, forgive me.*
> *Thank you.*
>
> *I love you." (3x)*

This mantra is part of the ancient *Hawaiian Ho'ponopono* method which entitles recognizing the past, even one's mistakes, is the first step to heal. Please note that this mantra has to be repeated out loud 3 times. Use it whenever bad feelings or thoughts arise to your mind to stop them. In this way you will heal inside and you will see how your mind and energy changes after reciting them.

When you finish the meditation, be thankful for the work done revisiting and recognizing your past experiences, and then work on forgiving yourself for whatever happened because you did the best you could do. Give yourself love and appreciation and be proud of your braveness for opening painful wounds and stop avoiding them. Believe me, this is the only way that you will be able to heal once and for all.

Become accepting and compassionate

As you meditate through your experience, try to understand it and empathize with it. It the idea I just gave to you with the mantra. This allows you to be compassionate towards yourself and ease of your emotional challenges when they arise. This helps you to understand the past experience, accept what happened, and forgive yourself for it. The forgiveness is very important because most of the time we are not guilty for what happened to us be we feel so, that it is why it is good that you forgive yourself even if it was not your fault.

Take a break, it is important

It is not easy to face your pains and fears. In fact, it takes great courage that is way you have to do cautiously to avoid becoming overwhelmed. Pay attention to each experience and do not rush through. When you feel overwhelmed by emotions, it is advisable to take a break. When you feel better, you can resume. The key is to increase your self-awareness to a tolerable pace.

Calm yourself

To soothe yourself, take a relaxing bath, go for a walk, cook your favorite food. Later I will explain you how to earn how to breath mindfully focusing, on how to inhale and exhale because it helps you to bloc other feelings.

Bring it all together

Realize that to heal yourself start by healing your past experiences. Recognize the pain, accept it, and be compassionate towards it. You will notice that you start developing a deeper self-awareness and understanding over the experience while increasing your tolerance around it. As you progress, learn to recognize when you are approaching the limit of what you can handle and calm yourself down at that point. Remember to always be grateful and loving to yourself. This deep inside work can't change your past or what happened to you, but it will surely change the way you experience that past incident allowing you to forge forward stronger and liberated with a more positive attitude towards life.

It is important to investigate every area of your life, to known yourself and declutter your mind from any burden in order to heal. In this chapter I have explained you how your past affects your life today, your thoughts and your actions. Until now you have learned different techniques you can use to investigate your past and find healing because is the only way to find your true self and live a better life. Not all techniques are good for everyone that is why you will have to find yours, and to do so, you can only try. Start with the exercises because even if they seem obvious or stupid I can assure that they work. The mind loves playing games and it gets lost in them so if you find a way to distract your mind from the ego and your solidified unconscious patters by recognizing them, then you get rid of any burden of procrastinating feelings and thoughts that are holding you down. Explore and cure your phobias, fears, addictions if any, and give yourself peace of mind. Always remember to inform yourself and engage a trusted professional to guide you through the technique you will choose.

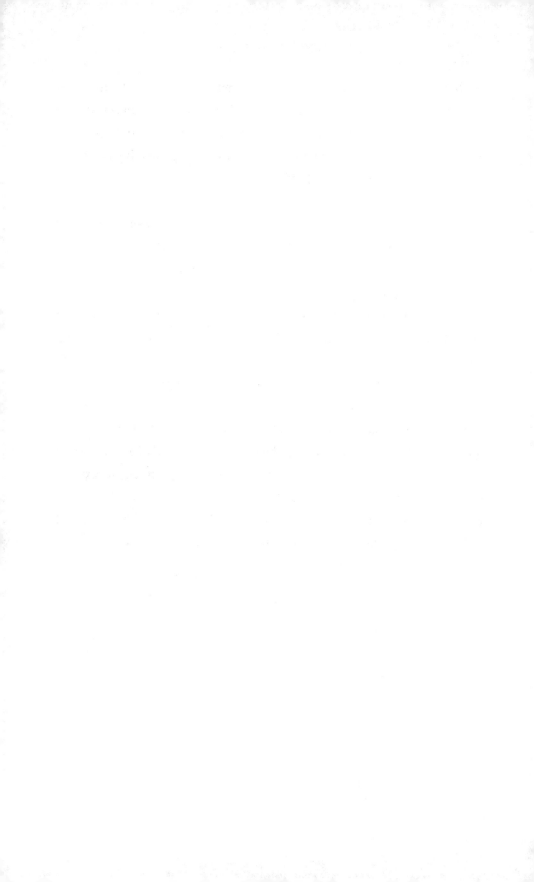

CHAPTER FOUR

THE POWER OF YOUR MIND

I f you have reached this chapter of the book, you understand by now that our brains have hidden depths that unconsciously but directly influence our lives. But as I have also explained, our minds are surprisingly open to manipulations that can change us for the better. Whether it's psychological tricks that change our long-term behaviors, hypnosis or new methods with healing powers, it can be made.

The power of the mind is among the strongest powers and most useful once understood and used for the self-wellbeing. The power of your mind comprises your thoughts, your desires, your habits, your fears, blockages and all your anxieties. The thoughts that dominate your mind usually influence your attitude and behavior and likely control your reactions and actions towards situations. This is why is so important to be aware of their origins and causes and where they may take you your thoughts. The majority of human beings like routine and are stuck in their ways, because as I explained you before, our mind and the Ego are not interested in any change or any effort that will take them out from the comfort zone.

If you are stuck in the same old rut, failing to reach your goals, then you need to do the right switch in your mind to change things for the better. Habits are defined as actions performed routinely in certain contexts and situations, often unconsciously and our mind is very attached to its own routine and hates changes. You have to realize that habits rule your daily life and only understanding how they are stuck in your thoughts will help you to nail the habits you want to keep and drop the ones that are blocking you. Old habits die hard, but the die. It will require effort to break the way your mind works your thought system. It is said that it takes 21 days to form a new habit or get rid of an old one.

This power of the mind is very creative and it is possible to train and strengthen it. Your thoughts come from your conscious mind and travel to your unconscious mind Like seeds, thoughts naturally grow and manifest in your life if fed with enthusiasm, attention, and interest, then your actions are influenced by this. Your thoughts also can influence the minds of other people. People in a position to help may find themselves helping you without understanding why.

You have to take care to feed and stimulate your brain in order to expand your mind. The two are inextricably connected. The brain is the equivalent of a human supercomputer and maximizing its ability is essential to becoming the success you want to be. The two together control who you are, how you think, feel and act. But is where all your potential lays and you have the incredible opportunity to go as far as you desire once you break your barriers. You need to change the beliefs that are stopping you from becoming who you are meant to be. Start believing in yourself and that you can do anything you set your intention to. Know that it will require effort and you may have to changes many things in your present life but if you are determined you will reach your goals. For example: If you want to lose weight of get fit, just wake up an hour before you usually do and go for a walk or a run. That will probably affect also the time you go to bed, so you can get a good rest of 8 hours. Believe that you can do it and do listen to your mind when in the morning it starts procrastinating you, thinking that it is too cold, dark or that you can start tomorrow, just ignore those thoughts and do it. Nothing can stop you if you have the right mid setting. Always pay attention to your thoughts, try to reject negative thoughts and focus only on thoughts that are constructive and may bring you positive results.

> *"If you have a strong mind and plant in it a firm resolve, you can change your destiny."*
>
> *Paramahansa Yogananda*

In this chapter I will explain you the hidden powers of your mind and how practicing the exercises explained, you may increase the understanding and the power of your mind.

Shaolin Monks

The Shaolin monks are a good example of what we can do if we strive and develop our mind. They believe that all strength comes from the mind and that when you train your mind, there are no limits to what the human body can do and endure. Through meditation, the Shaolin monks have been able to control energy and perform extraordinary feats. They have been known to use intense concentration to endure pain and channel energy in order to push their bodies to the limit. Deep concentration allows them to master and control their 'CHI' which is the vital force that forms part of any living entity, the flow of which must be balanced for good health. This controlling of their chi through the mind makes them temporarily immune to pain and enables them to perform these feats that seems impossible.

While Shaolin monks seem to achieve the unimaginable, they have simply developed their minds and bodies in ways that allow them to perform extraordinary feats of mental and physical strength by tapping into their internal energy and through physical conditioning. These monks are able to actually raise their body temperatures with their minds and dry wet sheets that are wrapped around their cold, naked bodies. They use meditation to endure pain and take one's mind away from the source of pain, for example, focusing the mind on other parts of the body. To combat discomfort, they also train in breathing and relaxation. All these feats that seem extraordinary can be achieved through the power of the mind through meditation and the control of the chi. This show us that the mind can be changed and that is a very powerful tool once you learn how to use it for your own good and redirect it to achieve any goal you set.

Keys to unlock your power of the mind

- Take time to stimulate your brain, and you will realize that you will be expanding your mind too. Focus on maximizing its potential and you will be on the way to success.
- Learn new skills to keep your brain engaged and challenged. This allow your brain to build new neural connections and improve your cognitive functions. Learn a new language, engage in workshops and new hobbies or activities like martial arts, dance.
- Be curious and constantly question things even if they seem obvious or basic. Don't accept what you are told.
- Read as reading engages your imagination and is an excellent way to learn new things and to learn to see people, places, things, and ideas in new and different ways. It will also improve your vocabulary and provide you with new ideas and points of view.
- Play with your brain to keep it awake and fit. Play games or do puzzles. You can find them online and as smartphone apps.
- Write things down as it helps new information to be easier integrated in the brain.

- Do not forget to feed your brain with foods that contain high amounts of omega-3 fatty acids, like walnuts and fish; foods rich in magnesium; antioxidant-rich foods like blueberries, blackberries, plums, red beans or black bean and plenty of whole grains like oatmeal, brown rice, and oat bran. It is important that you exercise regularly because cardio activity releases a potent mix of hormones important to improving mood, relieving stress, and boosting concentration and get enough sleep at least 6-8 hours each night.

UNDERSTANDING THE THIRD EYE

The third eye is also called the mind's eye or inner eye because it provides perception beyond ordinary sigh. Buddhism and Hinduism use it as a symbol of enlightenment and they refer to it as the eye of knowledge, the gateway to greater consciousness.

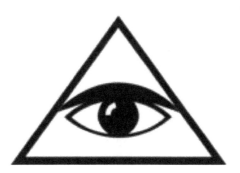

It is an invisible eye which refers to the gate that leads to inner realms and spaces of higher consciousness. Positioned between the brows and just above the eye level, the third eye is associated with intuition and wisdom. In the human body, this energy center is traditionally associated with the pineal gland. Note that body glands and chakras are intimately related as they represent different levels of bodily functions, the first one being focused on the physical, the other on the subtle energetic level. The third eye is located on the forehead, between the eyebrows slightly above at the bridge of your nose. It is the center of intuition and foresight. Contrary to a common misconception, it is not located in the middle of the forehead, but between the eyes where the eyebrows would meet. The function of the third eye chakra is driven by the principle of openness and imagination. The Third eye chakra or Ajna (which means "command" and "perceiving") is associated to the pineal gland in charge of regulating biorhythms, including sleep and wake time. The pineal gland is located in the middle of the brain, at the same level as the eyes. This gland is usually considered to be in charge of producing melatonin and regulating our sleep cycle and our sexual maturation. The ways it functions is closely connected to the cycles of light and darkness.

The third eye is an instrument to perceive the subtler qualities of reality. It goes beyond the physical senses into the realm of subtle energies. Awakening of the third eye allows you to open up to an intuitive sensibility and inner perception. The third eye chakra is associated with characteristics such as vision, intuition, perception, psychic abilities (clairvoyance and clairaudience), connection to wisdom and insight, and inspiration and creativity. It connects us with a different way of seeing and perceiving and puts us in touch with the ineffable and the intangible more closely. Third eye visions are also often subtler than regular visions as they may appear blurry, cloudy, or dream-like.

Note that we are all born with the third eye, but to start using it you will need to become aware of it and practice to develop its potential. Sustaining awareness of third eye chakra energy might require focus. When we focus our mind and consciousness, we can see beyond the distractions and illusions that stand before us and have more insight to live and create more deeply aligned with our highest good.

There are several things you can try to awaken your third eye as the following:

- Exercise your intuition
- Guided meditation, silent meditation
- Let your imagination loose
- Pay attention to your dreams
- Try doing visualizations
- Commune with nature and the energy of the elements
- Start a creative craft
- Try to free flow
- Practice contemplation
- Cultivate your psychic abilities

Let me show you how you can help to develop some of the third eye abilities.

Intuition

Intuition can be described as a process that will give you knowledge about something without analytic reasoning. Intuition bridges the gap between the unconscious and the conscious parts of your mind, as well as between reason and instinct. A person needs both instinct and reason to enable them to make the best decision regarding any aspect of their lives.

Intuition is a build-up of experiences, instincts and senses, which includes heightening the touch, feeling, sight, hearing, and taste to its very peak. Intuition comes from the observation of one's own mental and emotional processes. It is your ability to sense things before they hit you. You may not know exactly why or have any logical reasoning for feeling that way, but at that very moment, you know that you have to listen and to trust that overwhelming feeling. For example, when you meet someone for the first time and shake hands, you may intuitively sense through touch and sight that you can or can't trust this person. This could be an intense feeling, because in your heart and gut you know that something is right or wrong. You can perceive a warm feeling of inner peace and love in your heart, or you can feel danger. Although we receive messages in different ways, we all receive them, even if we are not tapping into them. Some of us feel things, while others see or hear them.

Be careful not to mistake intuition for fear or anxiety. It can be confusing and it's important to know the difference. Intuition can be recognized as an inner guidance, a kind of knowing, or you might say an internal compass: a hunch, a gut feeling, or an instinct would describe the way intuition influences our behavior. On the other hand, a negative emotion, will express itself through a physical response such as aggressiveness, sweating, an adrenaline rush, or a racing heart. The difference between them is that fear will lead to take a decision that makes you feel relieved, as though you just survived a threat while intuition will lead you towards a more path comfortable, even if we are not certain. Understanding the difference is important if we really want to properly access our intuition.

Before you can improve access your intuition, you first have to be able to hear it within the noise of your busy life Note that you should not try to use your intuition when using your head, meaning thinking too much, because then you'll be using your ego and your intuition will not be able to come through. Use your intuition when you are calm and not rushed.

Here are some methods to improve access to your intuition:

Practice Mindfulness

Mindfulness means to focus on being in the moment. Mindfulness is a great technique to filter out all the distractions in your environment and your brain because only a quiet mind is able to hear intuition over fear.

Trust your gut

The gut is lined with a network of neurons and it's often referred to as the "second brain". I will develop this idea in a separated chapter, but for now, know that the gut is nervous system that contains around 100 million neurons. This is why you feel "sick" when having to make a tough decision or knowing you've made a bad one. Pay attention and listen to our intuition trusting your guts.

Be aware of your dreams

Dreams are packed with valuable information such as learnings, experiences, and memories. Paying attention to our dreams can provide information that we may not have access when we are awake. Therefore, before going to sleep, it's essential for you to direct your thoughts to any unresolved issues and think about possible options or solutions as you're falling asleep. Close your eyes and let your brain do the rest. Keep a notebook close to your bed and write what you have dreamt the first thing in the morning when you still remember your dreams. Try to be as detailed as you can in journaling your dreams because it will help you to improve your memory and get the messages you need to know.

Intuition is developed from the third eye. Practice the following exercises to understand how intuition works. If you keep on practicing them, it with strengthen this ability.

Exercise 1

Take a deck of cards and spread it on a table with the cards looking down. Take three deep breaths to clear your mind and with your eyes closed, chose one of the cards. Put it in between your hands and notice how it feels. Is it cold? Hot? Maybe an object, a color? A Number? Do not try to answer these questions and do not force your mind. Keep your mind open and try to keep at peace, just notice your thoughts. The game consists of the first thoughts that come to your mind and note them. But do not think too much because when we start reasoning, we lose the intuition. Then open your eyes and check the card. Notice whether it has anything that was related to your feelings or thoughts while you were holding the card. Even the slightest thing is good because you are opening a sense that you are not used to using and it will get better with practice. Keep on practicing to increase your intuition sense.

Exercise 2

Take a plain white paper and cut it into 8 pieces. Draw a circle in each of the pieces and fill it with colors: 2 red, 2 blue, 2 yellow, and 2 green and put them back on the table facing down. Mix them. Take another plain sheet of paper and a pen. Take three deep breaths to clear your mind, take one of the papers without looking at it, and put it in between your hands. Try to guess the color by what you feel. For example, feeling cold in the hands could mean that the color is cold, blue, or green. Warmth could be yellow or red. What you think or what memories arise and try to guess the color. It has to be done without too much thinking, your mind has to be open and not judging your thoughts. Write your answer in the sheet and put the paper on the side. You will have to put the following paper under this one and so on in order to check the answers afterward and not get mixed. Then do the next one until you do the 8 pieces of paper. While you are practicing, your mind is going to come in between trying to make you reason how many colors are out and which colors you did not write in the sheet. Try to stop the right brain and let the left brain work. Once you have done the 8 papers, check the answers. Once again, remember that you are starting to use a new sense so the more you practice, the more you will understand how it works and your answers will be more accurate. If you wrote blue and you got a green, note that this is not a complete mistake because green is made of blue and yellow and is dark so you are getting closer. Count the right and wrong answer and try again. The only tip I can give you is that you try to stop the reasoning mind and observe your thoughts and all the information that gets to you. No one can explain or describe it, the intuition has to be awakened by oneself, and these are just easy tricks to do it.

Telepathy

Telepathy is the ability to transmit words, emotions, or images to someone else's mind. This kind of communication cannot be explained scientifically. It is usually the communication that happens between two minds that are separated over a distance and without putting into use the five senses. Everyone has experienced some telepathic moments in one way or another, for example: you may have been thinking about someone and get a phone call from the person—that is telepathy. It mostly happens between two people that have an emotional connection.

To understand telepathy better, practice the following exercise. Note that you need to relax your body and mind, visualize the receiver right in front of you, and focus your thoughts on sending a simple word or image. You need a partner to practice with, and you will have to take turns sending and receiving messages because telepathy goes both ways. Track your progress with a journal and with practice, you might be surprised to find you and your friend are developing this ability.

Exercise 1

To work on telepathy, you will need to practice with someone else to who you will be transmitting and receiving information. At the beginning you can be in the same room in front of each other. To make it easy, we will use the same exercise as in intuition. Take a plain white paper and cut it in 8 pieces. Draw a circle in each of the pieces and fill it with colors: 2 red, 2 blue, 2 yellow, and 2 green and put them back on the table facing down. Mix them. Now, sitting comfortably around a table in a quiet ambiance, one in front of the other, you both take 3 deep breaths to clear the mind and one of you, the transmitter, chose one of the papers that lie on the table facing down and look at the color. Now with your eyes closed or open, as you both feel more comfortable, the transmitter should try to concentrate on sending the information through the third eye to the receiver. Visualize it with as much detail as possible, and focus your mind solely on it. Concentrate on what it looks like, what it's like to touch it, and how it makes you feel. For that, the mind has to be free from other thoughts, just concentrate on seeing a wall of the color, and send it using the power of your thoughts. Please note that this is another exercise that requires practice to open the channel of transmission and to understand how to send and receive the information. You will have to practice being the sender and the receiver. Do not force yourself, be subtle in sending and getting the information. The transmission should not last longer than 3 minutes. In the beginning, try not to mix objects with the colors. For example, if you have red, just send red and do not look for strawberries, a red pullover, watermelon., etc., keep it simple. The person receiving the transmission should keep a clear and open mind and never make an effort or overthinking.

Exercise 2
Use the same method but try to practice using words, numbers, objects or geometrical figures.

You should find a subject to practice with that is open to the idea. Intuition and telepathy work as a telephone line; with transmitter and a receiver, and both need to have open channels. Remember that practicing these techniques means no thinking, no examination of your thoughts, no using your brain but your guts. Go with the first thing that comes to your mind without judging or giving it second thoughts. When the mind comes in, the intuition goes out.

POWER OF BREATHING: PRANAYAMA

Breathing is something that every living being does involuntarily as long as there is life. The first thing we do we are born is to inhale and the last one is to exhale. In yoga, breathing is referred to as Pranayama. This word pranayama is translated to mean control of life force or the extension of breath. Pranayama has developed in a formal practice of controlling the breath, which is the source of our prana, or vital life force.
Studies have shown that controlled breathing reduces the effects of stress

and enhances physical and mental health. There are different breathing techniques that aid in reducing stress, digestion, bringing calmness, and improving sleep. These breathing techniques are unique and are powerful to perform different functions in your body.

Breathing exercises

The following breathing exercises are basic but will help you to get in touch with your breath as well as help you calm down and find peace of mind.

Balloon Breath

This breath is useful to calm fear, restlessness, and worry. Lie down on your back resting your hand by your sides with your palms up. Inhale slowly through the nose and imagine you are filling your body with your breath and you are becoming like a big balloon. Exhale slowly, blowing the air out through your mouths. What is the color of your balloon? Do it 3 times.

Belly Breath

Is very useful when you are feeling sad or hurt. It gives self-soothe and comfort. Lie down on your back resting. Place one hand on your chest and the other one on your belly. Start breathing slowly and deep, feeling your chest and your belly move up and down as the air goes in and out of your body. Repeat at least three times.

Counting Breath

This breath helps to self-regulate and calm down as well as helps to gain clarity when feeling frustrated. Sit up comfortably, letting your spine grow tall. Take a deep breath in, counting silently 1...2...3...4...5. Hold your breath for the same count. Then let your breath out counting silently to 5. Try to keep the same rhythm in the three counts.

Breathing is a natural deed in all living things. It is also a very powerful tool that enables people to create ease and balance in their lives. Focusing on breathing will return you to a neutral state of being enabling you to feel rejuvenated, gain clarity, and improve your sense of being.

The following two breathing practices should only be practiced once you have tried with the above ones as they require some experience and more concentration.

Ujjayi Pranayama - The victorious breath

Ujjayi is particularly beneficial for calming the mind. It is known to be beneficial for those suffering from stress, insomnia, and mental tension. As I told you before, by controlling your breath, you calm your mind and bring awareness to the present moment. Its name comes from the Sanskrit word "ujjayi," which means "to conquer" or "to be victorious. When practicing *Ujjayi*, you completely fill your lungs, while slightly contracting your throat, and breathe through your nose. Because of the sound it makes when performed correctly, this breath is also sometimes called "Ocean Breath".

This breathing technique is used throughout Ashtanga and Vinyasa yoga practices in every pose because it helps to link your mind, body, and spirit to the present moment.

You can practice Ujjavi following the next steps:

1. Sit in a comfortable position and relax your body. Gently close your eyes and relax your jaw and your tongue.

2. Inhale and exhale deeply through your mouth. Feel the air of your inhalations passing through your windpipe.

3. On your exhalations, slightly contract the back of your throat, as you do when you whisper. Softly whisper the sound, "ahhh," as you exhale. Maintain the slight constriction of the throat on your inhalations, as well.

4. When you can comfortably control your throat during the inhalations and exhalations, gently close your mouth and begin breathing only through your nose. Keep the same constriction in your throat as you did when your mouth was open. Direct the breath to travel over your vocal cords, across the back of your throat.

5. Concentrate on the sound of your breath; allow it to soothe your mind. It should be audible to you, but not too loud.

6. Let your inhalations fill your lungs to their fullest expansion. Completely release the air during your exhalations.

Start by practicing *Ujjayi* for five minutes while you are seated. For deeper meditation, increase your time to 15 minutes.

The alternative nostril breathing

This is a more complicated way of breathing that requires practice and concentration. It helps to relax the nervous system and aid in sleep. This technique is believed to purify the blood, decrease stress, increase concentration, and calm the mind. It can be done while seated or lying down and can be done at any time. It has to be a relaxed way of breathing using one nostril at a time.

1. Find a comfortable seat. Come into Sukhasana (Easy Pose), or sit on pillow. Feel your sit-bones ground you as you create a long spine lifting ever so slightly from the crown of the head. Rest your left palm on your left knee, moving your right hand towards the nose. It is important that you keep your head, neck, and trunk erect, so that your spine is balanced and steady and you can breathe freely—a bent spine can disrupt your nervous system and increase physical and mental tension. Gently close your eyes.

2. Bring the right hand up to the nose and fold the index and middle fingers to the palm, so that you can use the thumb gently to close the right nostril, and the ring finger to close the left nostril. Be sure that you are not bending over to bring the head down to your hand and be gentle.

3. Using the right thumb, softly close the right nostril, and inhale as slowly as you can through the left nostril, then close it with your ring finger. Pause. Open and exhale slowly through the right nostril. Let each exhalation and inhalation be smooth, slow, and relaxed. Do not force the breath and let each breath flow without pause. Gradually increase the

length of your breath, but do not practice breath retention except under the careful supervision of a teacher.

4. With the right nostril open, inhale slowly, then close it with the thumb. Pause. Exhale through the left nostril. Once your exhalation is complete, inhale through the left. Pause before moving to the right.

5. Start by inhaling through both nostrils, then close one nostril and exhale and inhale smoothly and completely through the other. Make the exhalation and the inhalation of equal length and avoid any sense of forcing the breath. Now change sides, completing one full breath with the opposite nostril.

6. Continue alternating between the nostrils until you have completed a full round of three breaths on each side, for a total of six breaths. Then lower your hand and breathe gently and smoothly three times through both nostrils. Please note that when practicing three rounds in one sitting, the middle round begins on the opposite nostril, reversing the cycle of rounds one and three.

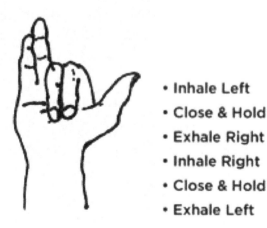

- Inhale Left
- Close & Hold
- Exhale Right
- Inhale Right
- Close & Hold
- Exhale Left

For a deeper practice, complete two more rounds. As the breath moves out and in through each nostril, it provides a quieting focus. Your nervous system will become deeply calmed, and your mind will turn inward and become steadied for concentration.

CHAPTER FIVE

AURA AND CHAKRAS

An 'aura' field can be defined as a luminous glow or radiation that surrounds a person's body, almost like a halo. Ancient depictions of religious and spiritual figures often feature this aura, but today, modern science is discovering that we are all, in fact, surrounded by this type of field, and it can actually affect the way we feel. The aura is usually described as an electromagnetic energy field. It is an oval-shaped ball of energy that surrounds your body. Some people call it the vibes that people emit.

The aura is found in seven layers known as the physical, astral, higher, lower, intuitional, absolute planes, and spiritual. Other people refer to the aura as the subtle body. These layers or subtle bodies exist around ones' physical body with each having unique frequencies that are interrelated. They affect people's feelings, behavior, emotions, and health. In case of a state of imbalance in one of the bodies, it leads to an imbalance in all the bodies.

Every plant and animal has an aura, and each one is as unique as a fingerprint. This natural energy field which emanates from your physical form serves a purpose. It can protect you and give you insight into those around you. If you happen to be at a concert surrounded by a big crowd of people you are exposed to a lot of aura intermingling. Your auric field connect and trade energy. That is why sometimes you feel tired after going to the shopping center or to a crowded event. The energy from your aura may join theirs and vice versa. As a result, some of your emotions rub off on them, and you get some of theirs as well.

Layers of Aura

The physical aura plane

It is the closest body to you and is decreased through your waking hours and increased as you rest or sleep. For the layer to be in balance, it needs physical comfort, health, and pleasure. People with negative space usually have a darker physical aura plane.

The astral aura plane

It is also known as the emotional layer and stores your emotional experiences. To know when it is imbalanced, you feel very sensitive, unstable, and irrational. To bring balance, it works well when you increase its needs with your surroundings like lie on the grass or sit under a tree.

The lower mental aura plane

This aura relates to reason, thought process, and constructing your reality. This plane is amplified when your mind is at work or focusing on a difficult situation. In this aura, your personal belief system is found, as well as your values and ideas. When this aura is imbalanced, you will easily get agitated, judgmental, and down.

The higher mental aura

This aura layer is connected to the lower mental aura layer but has a deeper spiritual element. Your higher mind beliefs like self-love, selflessness, gratitude are stored. Ensure this higher plane is always positive because everyone else can also sense the energy from it.

Spiritual aura plane

This solely deals with your spirituality and connects you to your immediate surroundings and the universe. When in balance, you can be connected to other people's spiritual layers too. If you have an imbalance of this, you will find that you are cynical, judgmental, and even threatened by your own spiritual growth.

The intuitional aura

This layer is also called the celestial layer. Your dream, intuition, and spiritual awareness are stored here. When in balance, you are peaceful, kind, calm, and patient.

The absolute aura plane

It works to bring balance and harmony with the other layers. It acts as a blueprint of your spiritual destiny and a store for all your experiences.

THE SEVEN CHAKRAS

Chakras are described as energy centers in the human body that help in regulating all its processes. There are seven chakras in your body from the bottom of your spine to your crown. Every chakra has a different vibration frequency, color, and controls specific functions that work to make you human. Chakras are defined as spinning colored energy wheels. The seven chakras are the conduit through which energy flows.

Blocked energy in the chakras can cause sickness, hence the importance of understanding what each chakra represents and how to keep the energy flowing.

Root chakra

Location: base of the spine / tailbone area: This chakra represents your foundation and a feeling of being grounded. It holds the feeling of being 'rooted' or grounded, your foundation and stability. Its emotional issues are centered on survival like finances, food, or money. Its color is red.

Sacral chakra

Location: lower abdomen about 2 inches below the navel. It brings the connection of acceptance of new experiences and others. Emotional issues linked with this chakra are: the sense of pleasure, enjoyment, abundance, sexuality. Represents creativity, sex and your ability to accept new relationships and situations into your life. Its color is orange.

Solar plexus chakra

Location: upper abdomen/stomach area. This chakra represents confidence, thoughts and feelings, and your ability to be in control of your life. Its emotional issues are related to self-worth, self-esteem, and confidence. Its color is yellow.

Heart chakra

Location: at the center of chest, just above the heart and it represents your ability to love and be loved, to enjoy what you love. The emotional issues linked with this chakra are self-confidence, self-esteem, positive mental attitudes and thoughts, self-worth. The color of this chakra is green.

Throat chakra

Location: at the throat. This chakra holds your ability to communicate clearly and to speak your truth. Its emotional issues are truth, self-expression, and communication. Its color is blue.

The third eye chakra

Location: on your forehead, between your eyes. It represents your ability to see the big picture, inner knowing, insight and vision. Its emotional issues are those of imagination, wisdom, and intuition. This chakra holds your ability to think clearly and make decisions. Its color is purple.

Crown chakra

Location: at the very top of your head (at the crown). This is your highest chakra, representing your ability Represents our ability to connect fully with our spiritual self. Its emotional issues are that of pure bliss, spiritual connection, and both inner and outer beauty. Its color is indigo.

Chakras

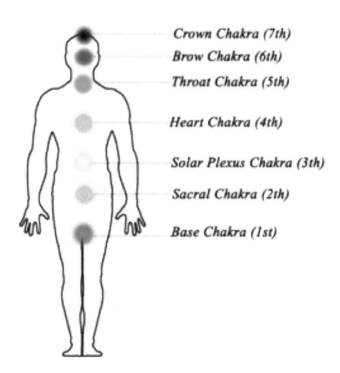

Crown Chakra (7th)
Brow Chakra (6th)
Throat Chakra (5th)

Heart Chakra (4th)

Solar Plexus Chakra (3th)

Sacral Chakra (2th)

Base Chakra (1st)

In order for our bodies to function in an optimal way, all of our 7 chakras need to be balanced and allowing our energy to flow smoothly through our bodies. If one of the energy centers is not functioning well, then the others won't function as well as they should. Some of them can even work too much or too hard (the third eyes over-thinking chakra is typical of this), which also sends our body and emotions into free-fall. Make a point to know your aura and understand the different chakras and how they affect your whole being. Work on the areas to improve after you understand the purpose of them in your life.

CHAPTER SIX

MEDITATION AND MINDFULNESS

'Once Buddha was asked; What have you gained from meditation? He replied: Nothing, however, let me tell you what I have lost: Anger, Anxiety, Depression, Insecurity, and Fear of old age and Death'.

What is meditation?

Meditation can be described as a set of techniques used to encourage increased awareness and concentrated attention. There are many forms of meditations and can be used as a psychotherapeutic technique or even as religious and spiritual practices. Most religions in the world practice meditation.

What is mindfulness

Mindfulness has been defined as the ability of a human being to be completely present, aware of where they are and what they are doing and not overwhelmed by the goings on in around them. It suggests that the mind is completely alert. It means being aware of every moment of your thoughts, sensations, and feelings. It involves accepting, thus paying attention to your thoughts without judgment of them.

BENEFITS

Better sleep

Research with adults suffering from insomnia and other sleep-related disturbances found that those that practiced meditation and mindfulness reported better sleep patterns and sleep quality.

Improved weight loss progress

Some people have struggled with yo-yo dieting in an effort to lose weight. Studies have shown that mindful meditation helps control stress eating and stabilize weight among the obese. Eating food mindfully was also found to help with weight loss journey, as well as support weight maintenance efforts.

Lowers your stress levels

Meditation and mindfulness help you learn how to control and minimize stress levels to your body and mind. This is important for your overall wellbeing. Studies have shown that mindful meditation improved mental health among the participants.

Decreased loneliness

Many older adults experience loneliness due to the loss of a spouse and also stresses due to medical issues. Studies have shown that mindful meditation over a period helps reduce loneliness and pro-inflammatory gene present in older adults.

Gets rid of negative feelings

Many people can go through a situation that will leave them feeling low and demotivated. Others due to the stresses of work may be affected health wise. Mindful meditation can help get rid of any negative feelings by focusing on the positive and helping your general wellbeing.

Improved attention

Brief meditation training has been found to enhance the attention span in people. It also improves your memory, reduces anxiety, and fatigue.

Management of chronic pain

Thousands of people suffer from chronic pain either from an accident or as a result of post-traumatic stress syndrome. Regular mindful meditation greatly reduces pain and helps patients cope much better.

Prevents relapse of depression

Mindful meditation is able to help a person disengage from dysfunctional thoughts that accompany depression.

Reduce Anxiety

Researchers have found that meditation can lead to reduced anxiety levels.

Increased brain gray matter

Mindful meditation has been linked with increasing the brain gray matter.

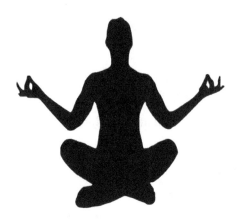

Meditation exercises for beginners

Exercise 1

Sit or lie down comfortably, close your eyes. Do not try to control your breathing, just do it naturally. Become aware of your surroundings, listen to the sounds and feeling. What are your thoughts? Focus your attention on the breathing and notice how your body moves with every breath. Do not attempt to control your breathing nor its pace and intensity. If you find your mind wondering, direct it back to your breathing. Maintain this practice for five to ten minutes and increase the time. Take it further and hum as you breathe out. Keep doing this and you will realize the benefits of meditating.

Exercise 2

Select a quiet place that you can comfortably walk to. Start by standing on one end of your path, let your hands feel free and comfortable. Open your senses and feel your immediate surroundings. After about a minute, focus on your body. Feel how your body is grounded on the earth. Focus and feel the pressure under your feet and other sensations, make sure you are present and alert. Start walking very slowly with a sense of ease and dignity and relax, paying attention to your body. With every step, feel the sensation as you lift your foot, then with mindfulness, place your foot back down. Concentrate on walking. When at the end of the path, pause, find balance, and carefully turn around. Pause again and become aware of your first step back. Continue this for ten to 20 minutes or more. If your mind wanders, return it softly. Repeated use of the walking meditation will calm you down and increase your alertness.

MANDALA MEDITATION

A mandala is a complex abstract design that is usually circular in form. In fact, "mandala" is a Sanskrit word that means "circle". Mandalas generally have one identifiable center point, from which emanates an array of symbols, shapes and forms. Mandalas can contain both geometric and organic forms that carry meaning for the person who is creating it. Mandalas represent the connection between our inner worlds and outer reality.

Designing your own mandalas can be both inspirational and therapeutic and can be used as a form of meditation, accessing higher consciousness, establishing a sacred space, and reflecting on the universe. The materials you need are just a piece of paper, pencils, pens or watercolors, even rocks, flowers or leaves to decorate. I recommend to start with a center point in the middle of the blank paper and move from it creating expanding rings outward towards the edge of your page. The less you think, the easier this practice of making mandalas becomes. Your mandala is *yours*, and you have the freedom to use your creativity to create a mandala drawing that is uniquely you. You do not need to have artistic qualities to do it, just try it and you will be surprised with the results.

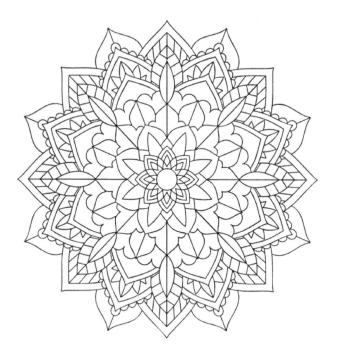

How to do it?

- Take a paper with a square shape. The square can be as big or as small as you like. The bigger the square, the more room you will have for putting in detail and color.

- Next, sketch out your own circular grid. To find the center you draw a straight vertical line that goes up and down, and a straight horizontal line connecting. Draw two more straight lines from corner to corner. Use your ruler and a pencil to draw a dot in the very center of the square and use the compass to draw circles around this dot. Continue making equidistant lines dividing the circles until you think is enough. By now you have something like you see in the picture below.

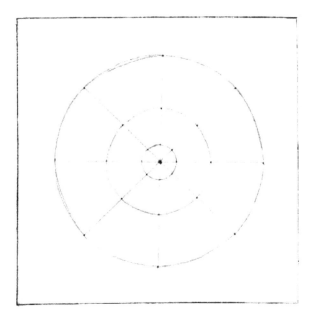

- Now that you've drawn the basic outline for your mandala, you can start drawing designs and coloring in the inside. Remember to always do it from the center direction outwards. That doesn't mean that you can no go back to the center and do new embellishments, but your work flow should start from the inside. Begin coloring the background of each circle and once finished and dried, draw the embellishments: circles, flowers, dots, whatever you feel like. It is important that you to repeat the patterns. For example, if you draw a star on one of the lines, draw it in the same spot on the other lines. Repetition is a key element in creating a mandala.

Drawing and coloring a mandala can be a highly enriching personal experience in which you enter in meditative state. The shapes, colors and patterns represent your current state of mind. Do not try to make it perfect or symmetrical to the millimeter. Do not put limits on how it should turn out, just let it flow and keep on painting until you feel it is finished.

Try it and enjoy the results of your art! If you want to examine your mind deeper, you can check the meaning of the colors and forms that you have used.

CHAPTER SEVEN

LAW OF ATTRACTION

The law of attraction is defined as the ability to attract into your life anything you are focusing on. Everyone is susceptible to the laws that govern the universe, even the law of attraction regardless of age, nationality, or religion. This law uses the power of the mind to translate what is in your thoughts and actualize them to reality. All thoughts have the possibility to become realty. If your focus is on negative thoughts, you will attract negative things and if you focus on the positive with goals to achieve, it will be possible to achieve them.

LAW OF ATTRACTION

This is the essence of the human power of the mind to create reality or in other words, creating reality intentionally. One of the most important writings about the law of manifestation is that of Kybalion. The book was published at the beginning of the XIX century under the pseudonym "the Three Initiates" and explains the teachings of a revered sage of the past, dated to old Egyptian times, called Hermes Trismegistus. The book is

113

referred to the mastery over the three planes of existence: the physical, mental and spiritual.

According to the Kybalion, there are 7 principles that are behind your ability to transform the world around you with mind power. These principles can be applied to a modern day scenario quite well. Keep an open mind and be willing to understand the core essence of its axioms from a universal point of view.

These principles are:

Principle of mentalism

"The ALL is mind; The Universe is Mental"

Everything that happens is a result of a mental state that proceeds it that means, that first is the thought or a design in your head, and then the manifestation of it into physical form in reality. The thoughts and images we hold in our consciousness begin to subconsciously manifest themselves in our external circumstances. The mind takes everything as it is because it doesn't distinguish the substantial from the real and the imagined (thinks about how you react when you are anxious or feel fear) and begins to re-create exactly that which we focus on the most.

The principle of correspondence

"As above, so below; as below, so above."

Everything in the universe and in all of the planes of existence (mental, spiritual and material) is connected and in correspondence. The macrocosm is found in the microcosm and vice versa. The solar system and life on Earth reflects the same thing on the cellular and atomic level There is a similarity between big and small events across the physical, mental and spiritual planes of existence. The outer world is a reflection of our inner world.

The principle of vibration

"Nothing rests; everything moves; everything vibrates."

All things in the universe are vibration and energy. For example, what we perceive as sound, is vibrating air that sends a frequency to the ears. This frequency is then translated into electrical signals that produces the experience of sound in the brain. In the same way, light vibrates too sending frequencies that are received by the eyes and translated into electrical signals, defining our perception of colors. These electrical signals themselves are a vibrating current.

Principle of polarity

"Everything is Dual; everything has poles; everything has its pair of opposites; like and unlike are the same; opposites are identical in nature, but different in degree; extremes meet; all truths are but half-truths; all paradoxes may be reconciled."

There is nothing like irreconcilable opposites. All polarities are degrees of each other. For example, we can only describe hot or cold as less hot or colder, take temperature for example: heat and cold aren't distinct entities or phenomenon but the same thing. Their only difference lies in the matter of degree. Also in the mental plane: fear and courage, love and hate are just varying degrees of the same thing. We feel them as different because of the different vibration, for example, love has a higher vibration than hate.

The principle of rhythm

"Everything flows, out and in; everything has its tides; all things rise and fall; the pendulum-swing manifests in everything; the measure of the swing to the right is the measure of the swing to the left; rhythm compensates."

This principle states that all things in the universe flow rhythmically. Plants may die but later will bloom, clouds will give way to sunlight meaning emotions can come and go. There is a rhythm between every pair of opposites and that this rhythm enables the transition from one pole to another. After every success there will eventually be some failures. For every action there is an opposite and equal reaction. The solution to deal with this rhythm is no to get attached to persons, places or material things, but to be always in the present.

The principle of cause and effect
"Every Cause has its Effect; every Effect has its Cause; everything happens according to Law; Chance is but a name for Law not recognized; there are many planes of causation, but nothing escapes the Law."
This means that every action has a corresponding opposite reaction. You can decide to be the cause or the victim of the effect. You have to understand the consequences of your actions and be responsible for them, so you will choose what actions to take, and, in so doing, you will also be choosing the consequences that will follow.

The principle of Gender and Mental Gender
"Gender is in everything; everything has its Masculine and Feminine Principles; Gender manifests on all planes."
This principle states that everything in the universe has masculine and feminine energy. Every person has a biological sex with a male of female physical body. However, psychologically, both qualities exist simultaneously in everyone.

These seven laws will help you understand the reality of the Universe and the power of your mind. I recommend you to read the Kybalion for a deeper understanding, but for now know that your thoughts can manifest into the world, for good or bad -that is why you have to be aware of them-, and that these principles can lead you to achieve self-mastery.

POSITIVE AFFIRMATIONS

The law of attraction would be a result of the combination of these principles. You can see it clearly if you put together the law of mentalism and the law of vibration. Using them together it will allow to manifest in the material world. Positive affirmations are sentences that you repeat often to yourself to build up self-belief in your subconscious mind. This in practice means writing down a list of sentences that motivate and inspire you to become better while helping overcome your inner barriers and self-doubt. In the beginning, as you recite these sentences, they may not be true but are designed to reflect what you want to be true. This consistent repletion of the positive affirmations will help mold your inner beliefs and the assumptions about yourself and the world around you. Based on the law of attraction, whatever you feel and think will shape your reality. Affirmations have the power to change your external world by changing your inner one at first. Note that your vibration around these affirmations is very important because if your energy is the same as what you want it will attract that vibration to you and you will get what you want. That is why it is necessary that you pay attention to what you feel when using the affirmation because without the right attractive vibration it will be useless. For example: if you want to go to Hawaii you should repeat the affirmation imagining that you are already there and feeling how it would be, so you will start attracting it with your vibration.

It is very useful to have a board where you can visualize your goals when saying the affirmations, so you have a clear mind of what you want to achieve and imagine easily the outcome. But first understand how mantras and affirmations work.

Mantras

Mantras are described as repetitive sounds used to get through the depths of the unconscious mind while adjusting the vibrations of all areas of your being. They are vibrated through mental practice, chanting aloud, or listening to them. For example, mantras are chanted during meditation or yoga because they help bring the concentration to the mind and clear the 'noise of the day'.

A list of positive affirmations

1. I have in me all the tools I need to succeed
2. My strength is greater than any struggle
3. I have decided that I am enough
4. I have the power to change
5. I am a winner
6. I will not take other people's negativity personally
7. No one can defeat me but myself
8. I am an achiever
9. I am comfortable in my own skin
10. I am proud of who I am
11. I choose to be positive, not negative
12. Happiness is my choice
13. I deserve good things
14. I have faith and hope for the future
15. 15. I have the courage to say 'No'
16. I respect and love my body
17. I accept myself unconditionally
18. I can do it and I will do it
19. I dare to be different
20. I am in charge of how I feel today and I chose happiness
21. I use my failures as a stepping stone
22. I am thankful for what I have
23. I believe in my skills and abilities
24. I set out to achieve my goals
25. I choose love over fear

Affirmations do not work by magic but due to the power of positive thinking. First, affirmations make you receptive to change, and then they assist in bringing the change about. This technic is based in the science of Neuroplasticity, the science of rewiring the brain for different thoughts. As we grow older it becomes tougher to change our thought patterns, but with conscious effort you can "rewire" your brain. One of the best ways to do this is by using positive affirmations.

In this chapter I wanted to make clear that you can get what you desire if you know how to align your thoughts and actions with it. Remember: all is mind. Use mantras and positive affirmations to attract the things you desire. Start by examining your life, see what you need and what you really want. Now that you know how the power of attraction works, write down some mantras or positive affirmations. Recite them every morning and see yourself transform your life. Come on and start now!

"Every day, in every way, I'm getting better and better."

Émile Couré

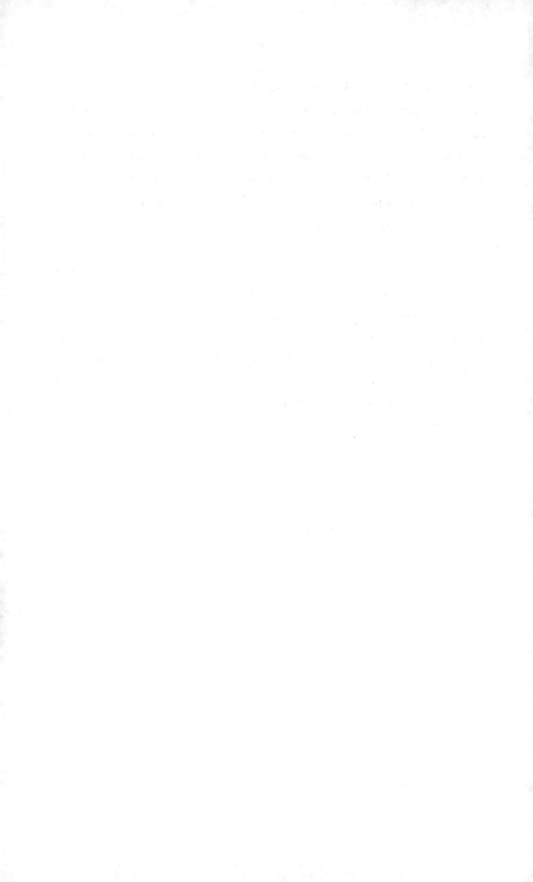

CHAPTER EIGHT

COLORS AFFECT YOUR LIFE

"If you wish to understand the universe, think of
energy, frequency and vibration."

Nikola Tesla

The colors we perceive in our environment originate from white light. The sun releases light at different frequencies and wavelengths that our eyes interpret as the color spectrum we see. The rays of color are energy and each color carries with it a different wavelength. The magnitude of energy in a single light wave is interrelated to its frequency. High energy is based on high-frequency light waves and low energy is based on low-frequency of light waves. When the frequency is high of color, the energy waves are closer together.

The rays of color are vibrations of energy forces that cover the globe and have a significant effect on our psychological, physical, and spiritual well-being. It is believed that each human being operates from a certain ray that is further influenced by secondary rays that are also known as the aura that surrounds living beings.

Every color correlates to different parts of the body, mind, and spirit. Color is known to influence moods. When you understand their effect, it gives you the ability to use the colors to influence your daily life, as well as promote your physical health and spiritual journey.

Red

This is the color of creativity, confidence, and courage. Our feelings are based on red. It is the color that promotes creativity, passion, and feelings of security. Those under red are courageous, spontaneous, confident, and are extroverts.

Blue

It is the color of spirituality and enhances your ability to see into the unknown. This blue energy governs the throat chakra. Those under blue are loyal and affectionate. Blue increases the energy for knowledge, clarity, and decisiveness.

Yellow

It is considered the color of wisdom. Most of the body systems are activated through the color yellow. It brings happiness, self-esteem, and clarity, as well as increasing curiosity and energy levels.

Orange

This color is said to increase the appetite for life. It is the color for the spleen chakra. It gives energy for life. Those under it are self-assured and playful.

Green

This is the balance of the mind and body. Like the color of nature, it is peaceful, compassionate, and loving. It is the color for those that want spiritual and physical growth.

Indigo

It is the color of the third eye. It is the color for those seeking for spiritual attainment, self-mastery, and wisdom. Those under indigo are idealistic, truth seekers, practical, and fearless.

Violet

Some of the worlds' most creative people are under the color violet. This color frequency governs the crown chakra and offers increased artistic creativity and talents.

The Law of Vibrations in Relation to Frequency

The Law of vibrations states that anything found in the universe, whether visible or not, broken down and evaluate in its most basic and purest form has pure energy or light that translates and exists as a pattern or vibratory frequency. All matter, your feelings, and thoughts have of their own vibration frequency. Every action, feeling, or thought that you choose has its own vibration rates. The vibrations will connect with what has a similar frequency. In other words, your thoughts are connected to the universe thus like will attract like. This simply means if you focus on good thoughts, good things will follow you and if you focus on negative thoughts, then negative energy will follow you.

For human beings, thoughts are where it starts. As you focus on certain thoughts in your conscious mind, they become firmly fixed in your subconscious mind. They now take the form of dominant vibrations and draws the thoughts to your life. In simple terms, your vibrations are the reason your environment is the way it is. It also affects the relationships around you. Your current feelings usually dictate your vibration. Your feelings are your vibrations. Negative feelings will result in negative circumstances and positive feelings to positive circumstances as they tend to the similar vibration.

Frequencies and properties of black, white, silver, and gold

The reactions to the color **black** are varied. Black absorbs all the light in the color spectrum. In some communities, it is associated with death and mourning. In ancient Egypt, it is a sign of life and rebirth and is used in fashion, because of its slimming property.

Color at its most complete and pure form is **white**. In psychology, it represents new beginnings. It is a symbol of purity, wholeness, completion, and innocence in most communities and even in psychology. It represents both the negative and positive aspects of all colors and has an equal balance of all the colors in the color spectrum. White offers peace and calmness. Provides comfort and hope. It is also the manifestation of the purity of soul and spirit, as well as thoughts. Is the color of fairness, independence and neutrality.

Silver is a metallic color associated with riches. It has the properties of gray but more playful, fun, and lively. Silver is glamorous, elegant, sleek and sophisticated. It is said to be the mirror to the soul, aiding you to see yourself as others see you. Silver also presents hope, meditation, kindness, mystic visions, psychic abilities, love, and meditation. Silver is also believed to draw out negative energy from the body and replace back positive energy.

The color **gold** is viewed as the color of extravagance, riches, wealth, and excess. It shares some of its attributes with the color yellow. It is a warm color associated with love, courage, magic, wisdom, passion, and illumination. Gold is also believed as a color that increases wisdom and power, aids in general wellbeing and health, lights the path to your goal, as well as creating success and prosperity.

Exercise on frequency and colors

Experience the colors. To know what a color means and the vibration it spreads is good to do it personally so you will know how it affects you and the others. For that, you will have to wear the color. Start with red, then blue, white, black, green, pink. You will have to be in the color as much as you can. Put on a red pullover, red trousers, and if you have red shoes. Wear for 2-3 days and notice how you feel and how others react to each of the colors. Please do not mix colors because at the beginning, it is necessary you feel one color by itself, plus mixing colors gives away another vibration and has another meaning. Have a diary and write down what you feel in the color and how you noticed the people reactions.

Frequency on the combination of blue, white, and red

Have you notice that most of the politicians wear a blue suit, a white shirt and a red tie? The combination of the three colors it is said to give the vibration of someone who is confident, serious and goal orientated, so is a good to wear these colors to an interview or a presentation. With a combination of the three colors, the energy you will send out is that of strength, powerful yet calm, trustfulness, and stability.

Wearing different colors leaves different impressions. The choices of color you combine usually gives out different things about your personality. Red is a strong and captivating color that indicates energy, strength, and power. If you have a need to draw attention to yourself, wear red. Blue color, on the other hand, is calm and relaxing. When you put on a blue color, it gives the impression of loyalty and trust. White is the color that reflects purity and innocence. In most cultures, it is the color used for brides. White is often associated with goodness and peace.

Colors affect your mood and that of the others who are in contact with you because you are sending out a vibration even if you are unaware of it. The choice of colors, of your dressing accessories and make up will reflect your personality and the impression you give to others. Try to choose colors that lift you up when you are down, vibrate according to your goals and release the image of your authentic personality. Try it! You will be surprised.

CHAPTER NINE

ASTROLOGY AND HOROSCOPE

"As above, so below; as below, so above."

The Kybalion

Since the beginning of times, most human civilizations like the Babylonian, Indian, Chinese, Egyptian, Celtic and Inca, among others, based their culture on complex systems of astrology, which provided a link between the cosmos with the conditions and events on earth. By then, the astrological practice was not understood as a mere divination because it also served as the foundation for their spiritual culture and knowledge-systems. They used that knowledge for practical purposes such as the creation of calendars and even contributed to the development of astronomy as the study of the skies provided invaluable insights about celestial bodies.

Thanks to these observations our ancestors could predict tides and eclipses, and were able to list some of the planets in the solar system and their movements.

Astrology has been defined as the study of the effects or influences that cosmic objects, like stars and planets, have on human life. Their position at the time of a persons' birth is argued to influence their personality and life. Note that the position of these objects at the present time affects you too, because they influence life on Earth. Most people are aware of their star sign which is in reference to the 12 constellations of the zodiac and use it to read the newspaper horoscopes which are too simple and too wide to refer to only one person. In order to produce better readings, you must check the position of each planet at the time of your birth creating a personal *birth chart*. The combination of planets, signs, and other elements like houses, will result in a more complex and accurate profile of a personality, future prospects, and life.

WHAT YOU NEED TO KNOW ABOUT HOROSCOPE

A horoscope is a forecast of a person's personality and future, typically including a delineation of character and circumstances, based on the relative positions of the stars and planets at the time of that person's birth. The calculations used are based on the date, place and time of birth. That's why a horoscope is so personal, like a fingerprint and the energies carried within it are unique to that individual. The planets, signs, aspects, houses, and other points reflect potential characteristics and patterns of a person, but free will can change these patterns and remodulate them for better. The horoscope shows our potentials and offers an insight and awareness about these potentials and their uses.

To understand Astrology, you have to first know that it is intertwined with Astronomy which provides the foundation and structure of astrology. Astrology uses astronomical, mathematical, and geometrical methods based on observation and correlation both in a scientific and divinatory manner. The observation and recording of the sky, the movements of planets and other heavenly objects by the ancients, allowed them to understand its effects on human lives and do quite accurate predictions as to their future appearances. They realized that specific heavenly orbs in certain positions would correspond to changes in weather or events in their lives, and noted these events as omens of divination for what was going to happen. Take for example how the moon affects the waters on the Earth guiding the tides and floods.

Horoscope is represented by zodiac signs that give you an insight about your life. The Zodiac represents the path that the Sun takes in our galaxy. There are 12 constellations, one for each of the signs of the Zodiac. Many of these constellations are represented by animals, like the Crab, the Ram, the Lion and the Scorpion, while a few are people such as the Gemini twins, and Virgo the virgin.

DIFFERENCES BETWEEN EARTH, FIRE, WATER SIGNS

The zodiac signs represent the sky's constellations having mythological tales originating from all cultures. Each one represents an archetypal energy of consciousness. There are differences but also many similarities between the signs as they all belong to the idea of astrology and the horoscope.

The four natural elements

The 12 zodiac signs belong to one of the four elements: Air, Fire, Water and Earth. These elements represent an essential type of energy that acts in each of us. Each of these groupings have unique traits, but they are interdependent of each other forming the natural world. Note also that each sign expresses that fiery, watery, earthy or airy temperament in a different way.

Fire

Fire signs comprise of Aries, Sagittarius, and Leo. They tend to be passionate, dynamic, and temperamental. They get angry quickly, but they also forgive easily. They are adventurers with immense energy. They are usually physically very strong, intelligent, self-aware, and idealistic, always ready for action. They burn out quickly without fuel to keep going, but can equally regenerate its power from ashes. A spark can set off a huge fire and as a result, these signs need careful management and nurturing.

Air

Air signs are Gemini, Libra, and Aquarius. These represent the mental energies within us. They are about ideas, motion, and action. They are rational, social, and love communication and relationships with other people. They are thinkers, friendly, intellectual, communicative and analytical. They love discussions, social gatherings and books. They enjoy giving advice, but they can also be very superficial.

Earth

The earth signs comprise of Taurus, Capricorn, and Virgo. They are realistic and firmly grounded and often bring people down to earth. They are faithful through all times to people. They are mostly conservative and realistic, but they can also be very emotional. They are usually practical, loyal and stable and can be very stubborn. They have diverse traits of being practical and on the negative, they can be materialistic and superficial.

Water

The water signs comprise of Scorpio, Cancer, and Pisces. They are extremely sensitive, intuitive, and emotional. They are mysterious and unpredictable. They can also be very refreshing and easily drown people into their depths. They usually have intense dreams that are almost psychic. They value security.

THE TWELVE ZODIAC SIGNS

Each sign has its own strengths and weaknesses, its own specific traits, desires and attitude towards life and people.

Aries (March 21 - April 20)

Aries are initiative, courageous, impulsive, and determined. They are competitive and highly dynamic. Aries is ruled by Mars the god of war and aggression, energy and drive. Arians are highly impatient and competitive. They like to feel strong like a hero–or to be swept away by one. As the zodiac's first sign, they were born to be number one and can inspire others with their confidence. They can a little bossy and get angry when they don't get things their way. They are adventurous and born leaders but they have to learn to let other people be the boss every now and then, and focus their competitive streak into worthy goal.

Taurus (April 21 - May 20)

Taurus are stable, loyal, clever, practical, and artistic. They have a perseverance personality. Taurus is ruled by Venus, the planet of love and beauty. They love great food, romance and beautiful things. They seek security and enjoy earthly pleasures. Taurus are hard workers but can operate at two speeds: either totally relaxed, or charging headfirst towards a target. They want to be comfortable, and surrounded by life's finest offerings. The can become very stubborn and don't change unless they see a really good reason in it, that is why they have to be careful not to get stuck and become stagnant. Taurus should learn to take new chances and sometimes risk in life as it can bring the progress and reward they are wishing for.

Gemini (May 21 - June 20)

Open minded, strong leadership qualities, kind, and ambitious. They like being involved and are curious. Gemini is ruled by Mercury, the planet of communication, technology and the mind. They are very curious, adventurous and very changeable. They have at least two personalities inside and constantly flip between moods and interests. Their mind is fast moving and they can get bored easily. They hate feeling stagnated and need continually new ideas and horizons being it at work, love or life in general. They should learn to stick to their goals for the long haul. They love to chatter, technology and gadgets and have a million great ideas. They have to watch their temptation to gossip.

Cancer (June 21 - July 22)

They are tenacious, generous, family oriented, and honest. They are faithful and expect nothing in return for their generosity. Cancer is ruled by the Moon, and their moods go through many cycles. They are sensitive, intuitive and nurturing, even psychic. Cancers are family oriented and like domestic life. The can get moody, and on that occasions they should be comforted, or else just left alone. They hate feeling threatened or vulnerable and will pinch others when so. With age they learn to control their feelings and moods.

Leo (July 23 - August 22)

It has the traits of humor, warmth, passion, joy, pride, and generosity. The Sun is the center of the solar system and the ruler of Leo. Leo is the sign of drama, but also a natural-born leader, who loves to be the boss. They need mega-doses of praise and appreciation. They think that the whole universe revolves around them that is why Leos should learn to be humble. They can seem self-centered but in reality they have a huge heart, and are very generous. They help and protect the people their love like a lioness.

Virgo (August 23 - September 22)

They are meticulous, mentally sharp, and methodical. They are perfectionists and great leaders. Virgo is ruled by Mercury, planet of the mind and communication. Virgos are detail-oriented, always analyzing everything, forming opinions and judgments. They may seem sweet and innocent, but their quick mind never misses a detail. Their work is usually impeccable. Virgo is also the sign of service, and are always there when help is needed. They are good listeners and give good advice. They are perfectionist and see every flaw that is why they can be too critical. They should avoid overthinking and learn to receive and not only give. They love the outdoors and should chill out in nature.

Libra (September 23 - October 22)

Libras are correct, fair, diplomatic, and romantic. This sign is ruled by Venus, the planet of beauty and love, like Taurus. Libras love to be surrounded by art, culture and beauty. They are smooth talkers, love good food and expensive things. They feel comfortable in harmonious environments where they show all their charm trying to keep everyone happy and engaged. Libras are social butterflies and like to be surrounded by people. They are fighters and they hate conflict and injustice and may get caught in the problems of others, but they need to remember to save some time for themselves and not forget to handle their own responsibilities and be organized. Libras struggle with indecision but their characteristic ambivalence allows them to navigate any social situation.

Scorpio (October 24 - November 22)

They are loyal, passionate, honest, and resourceful. This sign is ruled by Pluto, the planet of mystery, power and control. Scorpios are powerful and sensitive with a high intuition and concentration powers. They read people like an open book because they notice every little detail and pick up vibes from their surroundings. They can be very loyal and won't tolerate any betray. They are revengeful, jealous and naturally secretive. Scorpios should work on being more open to others and learn to develop trust to improve their relationships. Scorpios energy is strong and will go wherever the put it, so they need to be careful on their goals and avoid getting obsessed or possessive.

Sagittarius (November 22 - December 21)

They are friendly, sincere, ambitious and independent. They have a positive attitude in life. This sign is ruled by Jupiter, the largest planet in the solar system. Sagittarius are cheerful, free spirits, optimistic, confident, open-minded and ambitious. They love adventure and open spaces. They juggle a million projects, hobbies and friends. As the sign of wisdom and truth, Sagittarius are very honest but their honesty is not always welcomed. They should cultivate patience, and be careful not to come off as a know-it-all and work on keeping their promises and commitments.

Capricorn (December 22 - January 19)

They are patient, loyal, ambitious, very intelligent and professional. They expect privacy and respect. Capricorn is ruled by Saturn, the planet of tough lessons and wisdom. Capricorns are serious, play by the rules and follow tradition. They often see life as an uphill battle, with the ultimate reward arriving only through suffering and sacrifice. They are ambitious but patient and take one cautious step at a time. They are devoted to their friends and families, and always support them. Capricorns can stay strong through the hard times and take their word seriously. They need to remember to have fun too, and stop seeing life as struggle.

Aquarius (January 20 - February 18)

They are future-oriented, charming, inventive, knowledgeable, and loves meeting new people. They love socializing with friends. This sign is ruled by Uranus. They are known to be innovative and do things their own way, moving on a path different from everyone else's. Aquarius can appear eccentric because they have their own style; they love new ideas and have futuristic minds. They are highly individualistic and do things their way, but also an amazing team players. This sign is vibrantly social and loves to be among your people. They are hardworking and competitive when set for a goal. Aquarius can come out as a bit unsentimental on a one-on-one level, but they can be moved to tears by the plight of animals, the environment or other social justice issues.

Pisces (February 19 - March 20)

They are romantic, intuitive, compassionate, social, and artistic. Pisces is symbolized by two fish swimming in opposite directions. They are dreamers and their energy awakens compassion, imagination and artistry. Pisces have two sides and tend to use imagination to escape reality. Pisces are creative, love dancing, movies, poetry, and music. Their moods are mysterious, have intense dreams and high intuition. Pisces may feel helpless, but are much stronger than they think. They are compassionate and have healing powers. They easily feel guilty, that is why they should surround themselves with good-hearted friends.

This is just an overview of all the zodiac sings and their specific traits. You will need to go a bit deeper if you want to really understand yours because the influence of the traits may be different from one person to another depending in other factors like the houses in the birth chat and the degrees of the planets. I recommend you to do a birth chart, you can find lots of free pages in internet where to get it to have a first impression. An astrology birth chart is like a snapshot of the exact position of the planets at the moment you were born. It never changes and it shows the essence of your life path and essence. A chart reading can reveal your strengths and weaknesses, the opportunities for your growth, the best timing for your goals. To calculate your astrology birth chart, you'll need your time, date and place of birth. Try it and explore your personality to help you understand certain behaviors, what you need to cultivate and what you should avoid. Know your sign, study about it and the characters therein. Check the sign of your family members, friends and coworkers, and note which are the signs you have better relations with and the worst ones. Look up what their horoscope says about them. It will help you to understand your relations with them and even understand their unconscious behaviors. Astrology may not be considered a science but it has been used since the beginning of the times. Use it to understand your birth traits and become your better self.

CHAPTER TEN

EXERCISE AND YOU

"A healthy mind in a healthy body."

Juvenal

Physical exercise or activity is important as it improves your overall health and reduces your risk of developing lifestyle diseases like type 2 diabetes cardiovascular diseases. Physical activity improves your quality of life while giving you immediate and long term health benefits. Some of the benefits of exercise are:

- Decreases the risk of heart attack
- Helps you manage and maintain your weight better
- Reduces your blood cholesterol levels
- Reduces the risk of certain cancers and type 2 diabetes
- It helps lower your blood pressure
- Improves the strength of your bones, joints, and muscles hence reducing the risk of osteoporosis

- Increases your energy levels, hence improving your moods
- It gives you a healthier state of mind by blocking negative thoughts, increased social contact, and improved sleep patterns.

I guess that that you already know that sport is good for you. Now you have to understand that you have to really start moving, doing whatever you like, but move your body to improve your energy, your sleep and controls your thoughts.

What is "CHI," how exercise gives you more life energy
CHI has been defined as energy or life force and this life force is what goes low when you are sick and leaves your body when you die. When you develop your chi, you are likely to develop healing energy in your body both physically and mentally. In order to optimize your life force, you must develop your breath and physical exercises.

In ancient Chinese medicine, one of the causes of sickness is blocked chi. When your chi is at its optimum, you release energy and good health into your body. There are exercises and daily practices that help improve the flow of chi. One of the simplest practices is sitting in the correct posture. When your joints and muscles are relaxed and your posture is well aligned, your chi is able to flow. There are three main ways to improve your chi: through breathing, through physical exercise, and meditation. The Chinese practice Tai-Chi to uplight their chi. It is a combination of defense training, health benefits and meditation.

Walking as a form of exercise and its benefits
Walking is a form of physical activity that involves moving your body from one point to the next by the use of your legs. Just like any other form of exercise or physical activity, walking has many benefits. Some of the benefits of regular brisk walking are:

- Maintaining a healthy body weight
- Prevents the development of diseases such as high blood pressure, type 2 diabetes
- It strengthens your bones and muscles
- It improves your mood
- Increases your energy levels
- Improves your balance and coordination

When you walk faster, further and often, you are likely to experience more benefits.

Walking meditation

Walking meditation is a simple practice for developing calm, connectedness, and embodied awareness. It can be practiced meditation either indoors or outside in nature, such as after a busy day at work or on a lazy morning. Find a lane that allows you to walk back and forth. A place that is peaceful, where you won't be disturbed or feel observed. The lane doesn't have to be very long since you are just going to practice an 'intentional' form of walking. You will be retracing your steps. Walk 10-15 steps along the lane you've chosen, and then pause and breathe for as long as you like. Turn and walk back in the opposite direction to the other end of the lane, where you can pause and breathe again.

The art of walking meditation is to learn to be aware as you walk and open your senses to see and feel your surroundings. Try to do it and then bring your attention back to feel how your body is standing on the earth. Feel the pressure on the bottoms of your feet and the other natural sensations of standing. Let yourself be present and alert. Relax and let your walking be easy and natural. Feel each step mindfully as you walk. As with the breath in sitting, your attention will wander away many times. As soon as you notice this, acknowledge where it went softly and then return to feel the next step. Continue to walk for ten minutes or longer.

YOGA

Yoga is a spiritual discipline that is based on subtle science that aims at harmonizing the body and mind. It is both an art and science of healthy living. The practice of yoga results in the union of your consciousness to that of the universe, thus resulting in a perfect harmony of the body and mind, as well as human and nature.

Yoga practice is believed to have started at the onset of civilization. Yoga is believed to have originated thousands of years ago before the origin of any religious belief systems were developed. Shiva is said to have been the first Yogi and Guru. There are many benefits of practicing yoga, these are categorized as mental and physical benefits.

Physical benefits of Yoga
- Improves flexibility
- Improves muscle strength and tone
- Improved vitality, respiration, and increased energy
- Helps maintain a balanced metabolism
- Helps in weight reduction
- Improves your circulatory and cardio health
- Increases athletic performance
- Protects you from injuries

Mental benefits of Yoga
- Helps manage stress by keeping stress levels down
- It creates mental clarity and calmness
- Improves body awareness
- Reduces chronic stress symptoms
- Increases attention

Types of Yoga
There are many different types of yoga. With each style a bit different from

the others, you'll find variations depending on the teacher whether you want a more physically demanding class or an easy, relaxing, meditative class. I recommend you to try different styles and teachers before settling on one. Hatha yoga classes are best for beginners since they are paced slower than other yoga styles. Hatha classes are a first approach to breathing and exercises. If you are new to yoga, Hatha yoga is a great start for your practice. On the other side, Ashtanga yoga involves a very physically demanding sequence of postures. Iyengar style is really great for people with injuries who need to work slowly and methodically. In an Iyengar class, students perform a variety of postures held for a long time while adjusting the minutiae of the pose while controlling the breath.

- Hatha Yoga – it includes all types of yoga that are based in physical practice
- Iyengar Yoga – it is great for those working on injuries and joint ailments
- Kundalini Yoga – it is intensely physical and spiritual
- Ashtanga Yoga – it is also known as the eight limb path. It is very physical
- Vinyasa Yoga – it is developed from Ashtanga yoga, involves athletic yoga postures
- Bikram Yoga – it is done in a room heated at 41 degrees centigrade and 40% humidity
- Hot Yoga – postures are held in heated rooms
- Kripalu Yoga – it is more spiritually oriented
- Jivamukti Yoga – it is both physical and deeply spiritual
- Yin Yoga – it is slow paced
- Restorative Yoga – it is both relaxing and rejuvenating
- Prenatal Yoga – it is designed for pregnant women
- Anusara Yoga – the focus is on alignment

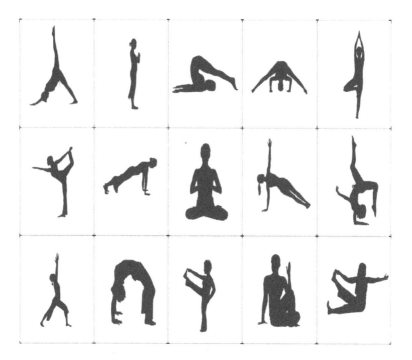

The Yoga Sutras of Patanjali

The Yoga Sutra of Pantanjali is the authoritative text on yoga. The message is that you must look within yourself for spiritual practices. That who you truly are lies hidden in the silence of your thoughts. That regardless of this fact, doubts, confusion, and chaos make you forget your true self.

The sutras further say that the hindrance to spiritual growth is stress that creates fatigue that leads to doubt and laziness. The causes to your suffering are forgetting your true self living from ego, clinging to pleasure and pain and the fear of death. This suffering will manifest as delusions that cause you to forget who you are, but when you commit to your yoga practices, you can overcome them.

Know that **the power of the mind is universal to everyone**. Learn to practice how to use your mind to your benefit. Learn the tricks to enhance your power and put it into practice. Take up the exercises discussed in this chapter and see how you can further enhance your mind power in dimensions you never thought before.

Exercise is very important for your wellbeing. Physical and mental exercises will go a long way into improving your overall wellbeing. Play tennis, football, jokey, go for a walk or ride a bicycle or take a walk, but move! Wake your body up and calm your thoughts. Try something new like karate, kickboxing, yoga, Pilates, something that you have never done before and enjoy the experience and the transformation that it will bring into your life. Remember that to have different results you have to start doing different things and do it. You mind will fight your initiative because it feels comfortable the way it is, but you have to step up and not listen to your thoughts but go straight for your goals and you will make it. Believe me, educating your thoughts is tuff but once you realize that you can do it and you actually do it, there is no way back to where you were. Include exercise in your life and feels the benefits.

CHAPTER ELEVEN

YOUR DIET

"Tell me what you eat

and I will tell you what you are."

Jean Anthelme Brillat

A ll living beings need food to survive. The food that you feed your body has been classified into 3 main categories that are the carbohydrates also known as the energy giving foods, vitamins the healing foods, and proteins the bodybuilding foods. Every food you consume will find itself classified into any of these categories. Food is another way we clutter our bodies with. In order to declutter yourself through diet, it is important to understand your food and how you relate to it.

Unhealthy eating is the way you get your body cluttered. Processed foods that are full of added sugars have become the easiest to access although the consumption of these foods causes many problems to the body, especially obesity-related problems. You need to intentionally understand your food, what is good for your body and what is harmful. Avoid careless consumption of foods especially junk foods and processed foods. Seek to have healthy eating habits to maintain your health and ensure your body systems function well.

The idea is very simple: if you feed your body with nutritious and good food, your body show it. You can even use food as a medicine eating what your body needs instead of what it does not need. The food you consume must be beneficial to your body as well as enhancing. Fruits, seeds and vegetables are basic for our wellbeing. For instance, consuming processed foods high in added sugar leaves your body feeling fatigued and you end up being less productive and feeling hungrier. Food has a direct relationship with the quality of life you lead.

The first think to do is to start eating clean. This term is being used a lot lately and it means cutting back on processed foods with refined grains, additives, preservatives, unhealthy fats and large amounts of added sugar and salt, as well as those that have artificial ingredients, such as certain preservatives and additives. Embrace whole foods like vegetables, especially the green ones, fruits and whole grains, plus healthy proteins (broccoli, tuna, lean beef, beans and peas) and fats (avocado, eggs, nuts, cheese, dark chocolate). All those substances pollute your body. It's about eating more of the best and healthiest options in each of the food groups, and eating less of the not-so-healthy ones Instead, the goal is to eat whole, natural foods. It also means to be aware of what you eat, where the it comes from, whether it has been treated with pesticides, and in case you eat meat or fish, try to understand that the suffering of the animal is also reproduced in that you later feed from. Animals that have been pumped with in closed in farm factories under artificial light and no space to move do not have the same properties (and vibrations) as the ones grown in their natural habits, plus may contain higher levels of antibiotics and hormones. I would recommend you to cut down on meat and fish and when you eat them, get a good quality bio product.

The practices of people with a healthy relationship with food are the following:

- Mindful eating
- Eat everything in moderation
- The timing of your meals matters
- They eat only when hungry
- They stop to eat when comfortably full, they don't stuff themselves
- They eat breakfast
- They avoid stocking unhealthy foods
- They portion their meals
- They are able to differentiate between snack and treat
- They allow themselves to enjoy eating
- They don't make up for missed meals
- They are not concerned about food to the extent of interfering with their lives
- They are not ashamed to be hungry

Food as medicine

Consumption of a diet that is rich in vegetables, fruits, and whole grains is beneficial to your body and mind. These foods help boost your immune system, provide essential nutrients like potassium, folic acid, magnesium, vitamins, and fiber which are vital for optimal functioning of the body. Potassium, for example, helps in the maintenance of a healthy blood pressure level. Dietary fiber is also essential in the reduction of cholesterol levels in the blood while folic acid aids in the production of red blood cells.

Food also can affect your mental health. Omega-3 fatty acids are also known to greatly improve mental alertness and concentration. The right food can protect against spikes of cortisol, a stress hormone. Food also helps trigger a hormone called serotonin that brings a feeling of comfort, hence comfort foods.

With a healthy diet, the body will be more resilient by building a strong immune system that will be essential in fighting infections. Diets that are high in legumes, fruits, fiber, vegetables, and some spices have been known to suppress the development of chronic lifestyle diseases. Nutrient-filled foods as opposed to calorie-dense foods are more filling and energize the body.

On the other side, foods that are highly saturated with fat and sugars contribute to obesity which increases the risk of developing type 2 diabetes. As you consume food, it is important to realize that food can be both poisonous and beneficial to the body. Eating the wrong food poisons the body in so many ways. Numerous studies have been carried out on people with chronic diseases such as blood pressure and the foods they eat, showed that once they changed their diet to a healthier one, blood pressure levels were greatly improved.

THE THREE BRAINS: BRAIN, STOMACH, AND HEART

We are used to think that we only have one brain, but is not so. Every person has 3 brains, the head brain, the gut brain, and the heart brain. The three brains are synchronized with billions of neurons working between them to bring harmony to your body and general health. In as much as these three brains work together, they also independently have different physical functions.

- The head brain is responsible for receiving information, analyzing it, and applying logic to it.
- The heart brain uses senses to understand the world through emotions and feelings.
- The gut brain helps us know who we are and our identity. It teaches how to follow instincts that are often referred to as the *'gut feeling'*.

For optimal health of a person, these three brains must function in harmony. A problem in one brain is likely to cause a problem with another brain, breaking the synchronized communication and harmony, hence causing havoc to your entire being. Ensure your emotions are in check, your gut is healthy so that the communications or signals that are sent to the brain to be interpreted are not misunderstood and are good for your overall health.

Importance of a healthy gut

A healthy gut is very important as they say all diseases originate from the gut. The gut is not about the digestion on, it is the second brain and as such has a lot of bearing to ones' overall wellbeing. The symptoms that are related to poor gut health include headaches, joint pain, fatigue, and weakness of the immune system. There are many benefits to a healthy gut to your entire being, these are:

- Improved memory
- Improved mood
- Helps build a strong immune system
- Hormone regulation
- Good digestion
- Improved mineral and vitamins absorbency
- Improved ability to eliminate toxins
- Improved mental health

The relationship between the gut and the brain

Researchers have recently discovered a lesser known nervous system in the gut communicates with the brain in our heads. These two brains are influential in the causing of certain diseases. For instance, some psychological concerns like anxiety and stress are also experienced by patients with gastrointestinal problems.

Gastrointestinal health has been linked to the cause of many sicknesses even mental and brain health. It is, however, possible to restore your gastrointestinal system to health because it is extremely important for your overall health including moods, memory, depression, and many more. There is a very strong connection between your brain and gut health. The way you think, your mood, mental health among others is linked to the second brain the gut just as it is linked to your brain. In the gut, there is the Enteric Nervous System (ENS) that is responsible for digestion. It performs its function to communicate back and forth with the brain about the general health of the gut as well as help build a strong immune system. For years, it has been known that gut health is connected to your mood. People suffering from bowel disorders, irritable bowel syndrome has been reported to be likely to suffer from mental diseases like anxiety or depression.

Probiotics and Prebiotics

Probiotics are good live bacteria and yeast found in the gut that aid in digestion and are good for your general health. Probiotics are nicknamed as the 'good' bacteria that are helpful in keeping your gut in good health. Probiotics can be found in the foods we eat that's why it is extremely important to have a healthy diet that includes foods that will produce probiotics in your gut.

Prebiotics, on the other hand, is said to be the food for probiotics. Prebiotics are a type of fiber. They are found in fiber-rich foods. Some of these foods include asparagus, apples, garlic, bananas, and onions among others.

There are foods that work against your gut bacteria hence damaging your overall gut health. In an effort to maintain a healthy gut, it is important to eliminate these foods from your diet. These will include highly processed foods that are high in added sugars. An example of foods to avoid include refined sugar, farmed fish and meat, gluten, soy, processed foods, artificial sweeteners among others.

What to eat for a healthy gut

To achieve a healthy gut, first, begin with your diet. What you eat determines the general health of your gut. Fresh fruits and vegetables are the best sources of nutrients in your body. They are high in fiber that helps in the increase of the good bacteria in your body. Consumption of fermented foods is also good for the improvement of your gut health. Some fermented foods you can consume include:

- Yogurt
- Sauerkraut
- Kombucha
- Kimchi
- Tempeh
- Fresh fruits and vegetables
- Whole grains
- Lean meats
- Low-fat dairy

All living beings need food for nourishment. However, what you eat and how you eat it will have a direct impact on your physical and mental health. Make a choice today to transform your life with healthier eating habits and in essence transforming your whole being.

Intermittent fasting

Intermittent fasting is not a real diet but a way of live. It is a timed approach to eating. Unlike a dietary plan that restricts where calories come from, intermittent fasting does not specify what foods a person should eat or avoid. Intermittent fasting has some health benefits, including weight loss, but is not suitable for everyone. At first, you may find it difficult to eat during a short window of time each day or alternate between days of eating and not eating, but after a few weeks you will get used to it.

There are several different ways of doing intermittent fasting. All of them involve splitting the day or week into eating and fasting periods. You should eat very little or nothing at all during the fasting periods, you eat either. Studies have shown that Intermittent fasting can have powerful benefits for weight control, your general health as well as your brain. It may help you reduce the risk of type 2 diabetes, heart disease and cancer, and allow you to live longer, with more quality of life. Intermittent fasting has proven to be also anti-aging as studies have shown in rats.

These are the most popular methods:

The 16/8 method

This method, involves skipping breakfast and restricting your daily eating period to 8 hours, such as 1-9 p.m. Then you fast for 16 hours in between. You can start fasting for 12 hours during the first week; then fourteen hours the next until you reach sixteen. It will help your body to adapt. Note that you may feel a bit tired at the beginning, but is only your body changing.

Eat-Stop-Eat

This involves fasting for 24 hours, once or twice a week, for example by not eating from dinner one day until dinner the next day.

The 5:2 diet

With this method you consume only 500–600 calories on two non-consecutive days of the week, but eat normally the other 5 days.

The worst mistake you can make is to compensate by eating much more during the eating periods. During fasting periods, you should only have tea, black coffee or water, but in case you break the fasting, do not worry, just try to keep to 16/8 most of the week. Drinking water during fasting periods is very important as it helps detoxing the body. If you decide to try Interment Fasting, I would recommend you to take some extra vitamins such as magnesium specially at the beginning. Many people find the 16/8 method to be the simplest and easiest to stick to. This diet allows you to eat without having to consciously restrict calories. But if you want to have good results, the healthier you eat the sooner you will notice.

CHAPTER TWELVE

RESILIENCE

*"Do not judge me by my successes, judge me by how
many times I fell down and got back up again."*

Nelson Mandela

T he ability of a person to bounce back or move forward after having faced adversity in life is what is called resilience. Resilience is about how well a person can adapt to events in their life. A person with good resilience bounces back quickly with less stress than a person with less developed resilience. Every person has resilience, the difference is how much you put it into use and how well you do. Having good resilience does not mean that the person does not feel the intensity of the challenge, but that they have discovered a great way to deal with it better and quicker than others.

Focusing on past experiences and sources of personal strength can help you learn about what strategies for building resilience might work for you. If you want to know how you usually respond to difficult situations in your life, ask yourself the following questions and think about your reactions to challenging life events:

- What kinds of events have been most stressful for you?
- How have those events affected you?
- To whom have you reached out for support?
- What have you learned difficult times?
- Was helpful for you to talk to someone else going through a similar experience?
- Have you overcome obstacles, and if so, how?
- What has helped you in hardship times?

Everyone has the ability to build and increase their resilience and it can be done at any age. All you will need is the willpower to do it.

How to build resilience

Developing resilience is a personal journey. People do not all react the same to traumatic and stressful life events. The following strategies can help you to build your resilience:

Make connections and have a good relationship with your friends and family. Learn to accept support and help from those that care about you. This will help build your resilience. Some people find joining social support groups helps them to build their resilience, go on, and join if you feel so.

Stop seeing crises as unmanageable problems. When situations come that are highly stressful, you cannot change them. However, how you react to them and interpret them will matter. Try and look beyond the now and how things will get better. Focus on the solution, not the problem.

Accept change as part of life. When you accept circumstances that you cannot change instead of stressing over them, you create room to focus on those things that you can change.

Focus on your goals and set realistic goals. Take small steps that steer you towards your goals instead of paying attention to tasks that seem unachievable.

Be decisive. When faced with a situation, take decisive actions, and avoid detaching from problems wishing them to disappear.

Seek self-discovery opportunities. It is possible to learn new things about yourself when faced with situations. It is possible to come out of the situation with better lessons, more spiritually developed, and with an increased appreciation of life.

Cultivate a positive view of yourself and trust your instincts and ability to solve problems, thus helping you build resilience.

Let everything be in perspective, even when facing stressful situations, avoid blowing things up.

Have a hopeful outlook. Optimistic outlook will bring positive outcomes. Focus on what you want not your fears.

Take care of yourself and focus on your own needs and feelings. Engage in activities that bring you happiness, thus helping you build resilience.

Ways to improve resilience

Find purpose in life, when faced with a tragedy, giving up is not the way to go. Find a sense of purpose like getting involved in community projects and so forth. This will improve your resilience and help you cope with the tragedy.

Cultivate positive beliefs of your abilities, be confident in your abilities to respond to crisis and improve resilience.

Create a strong social network, have confidants. Surround yourself with supportive people.

Embrace change and be flexible to change. This is a great way to improve your resilience.

Be optimistic and even when it is darkest, maintain hope. This is an important part of resilience.

Nurture yourself and take care of your need. Do not neglect yourself and the needs of your body.

Improve your problem-solving skills. People that are able to come up with solutions are better able to cope with problems. Every time you face a challenge, try to come up with possible solutions.

Establish goals, face the situations by setting realistic goals to deal with the challenge.

Take action to solve problems, you cannot wish the problem away. Take active action to solve the problem.

Keep working on your skills, building and improving your resilience levels may take time. Do not give up and keep working on your skills to improve your ability or resilience.

PSYCHOLOGY OF RESILIENCE

Resilience in psychology is called positive psychology. This is the ability to be able to cope with any situation that throws itself at you in life. People that get knocked by life and still come back stronger than before are called resilient. A person that is resilient navigates through challenges by making use of personal resources, strength, as well as psychological capital like hope, self-efficacy, and optimism. Relationships are key to building resilience. This is developed from an early age due to parental influence. Studies have shown that children brought up by authoritative parents were more resilient than those of authoritarian or passive upbringing. Authoritative upbringing is characterized by qualities of affection and warmth that give structure and support. Authoritarian style of parenting, on the other hand, often results in dependent children or even rebellious ones that often are withdrawn. Psychologists have formed the conclusion therefore that the style of parenting can affect the ability of a child to be psychologically resilient.

There are many factors that can affect one's resilience or ability to adapt to situations. However, regardless of your ability to be resilient, it is possible to build resilience or improve it in order to better cope with situations. This chapter is intended to help you with taking your own road to resilience. Focus on developing and using a personal strategy for enhancing your resilience when dealing with hardship. Being resilient does not mean that a person doesn't experience difficulty or distress. Emotional pain and sadness are common in all of us. In fact, resilience is learnt during emotional distress. It is not a trait that people either have or do not have, but behaviors, thoughts and actions that can be learned and developed in anyone.

Getting help when you need it is crucial in building your resilience. For many people, using their own resources (family members, friends, online resources, or books), may be sufficient for building resilience. At times, however, we can get stuck or have difficulty making progress. In those moments, can be helpful to turn to participate in community groups with other people struggling with the same hardships. In any case, it is important to get professional help if you feel like you are unable to function or perform basic activities of daily living as a result of a traumatic or other stressful life experience. Find someone you feel at ease with and work on your healing so you can move forward.

CONCLUSION

If you are already here, then it means you have gone through this book. Congratulations! This book has been written for you dear reader that is ready to start over and do it right this time. You have been stressed, confused, and even scared because nothing you do is good enough.

It is about time you took control of your life. Stop trying things and failing but know the secret of doing things successfully. Know that you may have to fight a battle more than once to win. With the knowledge you have acquired and the tools you have learned, you are now fully equipped to start a journey to your real self. Let go and declutter yourself from anything that has acted as an obstacle in your life. Now you have a sword in your hands to fight for your goals. This change is a lifestyle change and will not happen overnight, but with some effort and determination, you will start seeing and experiencing small victories every day. Why wouldn't you do something that for sure will be good for you? I assure you that knowing yourself, understanding your thoughts and taking care of your wellbeing will change your life for better and you can even make your dreams come true. Take the effort to do it. Easy said than done, but by all means, worth it! You are likely to face many challenges and sometimes you will fail. Do not despair, rise up and dust yourself to start a better life.

Always remember, this is an individual journey and so do not compare yourself with others who have made it, instead learn to celebrate your victories at every stage. As human beings, we are all different. The technique that may work for one person may not work for you. Personalize the journey and find what works best for you. Start now and find your path to true happiness, peace, joy, and love.

Do not let your mind

be the gap in your life!

Impressum

Alex Hollister

c/o Magdalena Mesquida Pujol

Stellinger Chaussee 6b

22529 Hamburg

Germany

mmp-ebooks@yahoo.com

ISBN: 978-3-949457-08-1

Alex Hollister

CPSIA information can be obtained
at www.ICGtesting.com
Printed in the USA
BVHW061249290621
610722BV00008B/809